Doulas in Italy

This book documents the emergence of doulas as care professionals in Italy, considers their training, practices, and representation, and analyzes their role in national and international context. Doulas offer emotional, informational, and practical support to women and their families during pregnancy, childbirth, and the postpartum period. Pamela Pasian explores the development of this "new" profession and how doulas are defining their space in the Italian maternity care system. While doulas are gaining recognition, they are also facing opposition. The book reflects on the conflicts and collaborations between doulas and midwives, as well as relations between different doula associations. Interweaving ethnography and autoethnography, it will be of interest to anthropologists, sociologists, and those working in health and maternity care.

Pamela Pasian is a postdoctoral research fellow at Ca' Foscari University of Venice, Italy and Professor of "Sociology of the Family" at the University of Padua, Italy.

Social Science Perspectives on Childbirth and Reproduction
Series editor:
Robbie Davis-Floyd, Rice University, Houston, Texas

This series focuses on issues relating to childbirth and reproduction from social science perspectives. It includes single-authored, co-authored, or edited books concerned both with people's reproductive experiences and with birth practitioners such as midwives (both professional and traditional), obstetricians, nurses, doulas, and others. It seeks to provide new viewpoints on functional and sustainable birth models and the challenges to their creation and maintenance, as well as on obstetric violence, disrespect, and abuse and their root causes. Single-case or comparative ethnographies on birth and other reproductive issues are featured, from high-tech conceptions to normal pregnancy and birth, including reproductive politics and human rights issues in reproduction worldwide.

Midwives in Mexico
Situated Politics, Politically Situated
Hanna Laako and Georgina Sánchez-Ramírez

Birthing Techno-Sapiens
Human-Technology Co-Evolution and the Future of Reproduction
Edited by Robbie Davis-Floyd

Negotiated Breastfeeding
Holistic Postpartum Care and Embodied Parenting
Caroline Chautems

Birth as an American Rite of Passage
Third Edition
Robbie Davis-Floyd

Doulas in Italy
The Emergence of a 'New' Care Profession
Pamela Pasian

For more information about this series, please visit: https://www.routledge.com/Social-Science-Perspectives-on-Childbirth-and-Reproduction/book-series/SSPCR

Doulas in Italy
The Emergence of a 'New' Care Profession

Pamela Pasian

Routledge
Taylor & Francis Group

LONDON AND NEW YORK

First published 2022
by Routledge
4 Park Square, Milton Park, Abingdon, Oxon OX14 4RN

and by Routledge
605 Third Avenue, New York, NY 10158

Routledge is an imprint of the Taylor & Francis Group, an informa business

© 2022 Pamela Pasian

The right of Pamela Pasian to be identified as author of this work
has been asserted in accordance with sections 77 and 78 of the
Copyright, Designs and Patents Act 1988.

British Library Cataloguing-in-Publication Data
A catalogue record for this book is available from the British Library

Library of Congress Cataloging-in-Publication Data
A catalog record has been requested for this book

ISBN: 978-0-367-76206-3 (hbk)
ISBN: 978-0-367-76207-0 (pbk)
ISBN: 978-1-003-16593-4 (ebk)

DOI: 10.4324/9781003165934

Typeset in Sabon
by Newgen Publishing UK

To Carlo and Adele

Contents

Figures

Foreword by Robbie Davis-Floyd

In the not-so-recent past, every time I used the word "doula" in formal presentations or informal conversations, I was often greeted with the question, "What's a doula?" This lovely and fascinating book answers that question with a detailed presentation of the development of the Italian doula and the multiple roles she plays in supporting childbearers throughout pregnancy, birth, and the postpartum period. Pasian's book is greatly enriched by her dual perspectives as both a doula and a sociologist, and by the fact that, rather than seeking to exclude herself from her research, she includes—even emphasizes—her own reflexivity and emotional engagement in her research process.

This book will be of interest to all those interested in doulas and the multiple services they provide, including social scientists, public health workers and researchers, medical workers, laypeople thinking of using doulas for their births, those who are thinking about becoming doulas, and doulas themselves in all countries—for, as Pasian shows, Italian doulas offer services that extend far beyond pregnancy, birth, and the immediate postpartum period to encompass the entire first year of the newborn's life. Thereby, they have created a model of doula care that doulas elsewhere might wish to emulate. For example, until I read this book, I had never heard of doulas who organize Blessingways tailored to the beliefs and values of the pregnant woman and her circle of friends, nor of doulas who help the postpartum mother with shopping, cooking, and other household chores up until the point where she feels capable of doing those things herself again. Pasian shows that in Italy, it is the mother who identifies the time at which such doula services should stop and describes the difficulties mothers have in letting go of the kinds of physical and emotional services that doulas in that country provide. I myself had a doula for my homebirth 37 years ago and was delighted by how seamlessly she resolved some tensions and disagreements that arose between my midwives and me, which stopped my labor until my doula, Rima Star, began chanting. Soon everyone present, including the midwives, joined in the chant and harmony was restored, allowing me to proceed to give birth to my 10-pound son. I never did let go of my doula—today, she is still my best friend!

Pamela begins this book with an interesting description of how the word "doula" became the name for this now-global type of caring professional, despite that word's still-negative connotations of "servant" or "slave" in the original Greek. She then describes how doulas developed in Italy, starting in 2007—much later than in many other countries—and the multiple doula organizations that now exist in Italy, the differences in the trainings these organizations offer, and the politics they must engage in to keep their practices legal. Pasian proceeds to distinguish between three ideological types of Italian doulas—the "progressive doula," who seeks to further the development of the doula profession, works politically to legitimize this new profession, and seeks to transform birth in humanistic ways; the "philanthropic doula," who sees her work as a calling to support childbearers throughout the perinatal period and aspires to a legitimacy based on the personal recognition of her clients; and the "individualistic doula," a charismatic figure who is often a leader in associations and trainings, and sees her doula work as neither a vocation nor a profession, but as a lifestyle that defines her essence and her identity. In contrast to their colleagues, these individualistic doulas tend to resist an institutional recognition of the doula profession as both unnecessary and dangerous for their freedom of practice.

Pasian shows us how, in spite of their differing ideologies, these Italian doulas—of whom she is one—manage to maintain a public face of sisterhood and solidarity, so as not to allow their intra-professional differences to interfere with the growth of the doula profession in their country. I find this overriding ethos of sisterhood and solidarity to be quite inspirational, as in my own country—the U.S.A.—doulas have engaged in bitter fights among their varying associations.

The fight around doulas in Italy, as Pasian shows, is not about the differences among doulas, but rather between doulas and the Italian professional association of midwives, which has resisted the development of the doula. While Italian doulas universally honor and respect midwives, and seek to work with them in harmony as supplementary helpers, many Italian midwives resent doulas because they take over the role of providing caring emotional and physical support that, according to many Italian midwives, should be the purview of midwives only.

During my (pre-COVID) travels to give talks, I have seen such midwifery resentment of and resistance to doulas occur in many countries and have watched these problems vanish over time as hospital midwives, who are usually unable to provide full continuity of care, come to realize the benefits of continuous doula care, and that they can leave the room to attend to their other patients with the comfort of knowing that the person laboring with a doula is well-attended in their absence. I firmly believe that hospital midwives, along with the laboring woman and her partner, all benefit from the presence of the doula, and that midwives everywhere should welcome, and not oppose, including the doula as part of the birth team. As Pasian demonstrates, some Italian midwives do support doulas and do appreciate the services they provide, most especially when they watch them provide those services in the labor room. And I hope that eventually, this appreciation on the part of some midwives will spread to all others, in Italy and around the world.

Robbie Davis-Floyd, PhD
Austin, Texas
1 September 2021

Acknowledgments

Books are never the sole work of the person whose name appears on the cover.

I first thank all the doulas who took part in my research, the doulas who encouraged and supported me, and the Italian doula associations' presidents at the time of my research: Emanuela Geraci, Laura Verdi, Chiara Pozzi Perteghella, Elisabetta Pace and Maria Chiara Purcaro, who accepted my questions and requests. In particular, I'm grateful to the Association Mondo Doula, which trained me as a doula and consistently supported my work, and the Association Le Lune Allegre, which surrounded me with a circle of supporting women.

I also thank the European Doula Network, in particular Debbie Mitchell and Maria Andreoulaki, for their help and kindness.

Among the doulas, most of all for their friendship, a superspecial thanks to Sara Cavallaro, Joanne Taylor, Valentina Vecchiato, Silvia Palla, and Beatrice Bosco for sharing reflection, laughter, and emotional outbursts!

My gratitude also extends to the midwives who took part in my research, for telling their stories and making dialogue both possible and accessible, among them a special thanks goes to Maria Grazia Biagini. Thanks to the National Federation of Midwives and the Midwives Boards of Belluno, Padua, Rovigo, Treviso, Venice, and Vicenza for their availability and hospitality.

I'm grateful to Tiziana Valpiana, Marina Toschi, Piera Maghella, and Maria Pollaci for sharing their experience and knowledge.

I'm also thankful to the photographers and friends: Beatrice Bosco, Sara Cavallaro, Marco Coltro, Valentina Dalla Pria, Alessia Galenda, Davide Lipari, Elena Luise, Silvia Palla, Joanne Taylor, Marta Tosetto, Licia Valso, and Valentina Vecchiato, who shared their photographs with me with enthusiasm.

Since this book is based on my PhD dissertation, many professors and colleagues accompanied me on this journey. I thank:

Franca Bimbi for her constant presence, generosity, trust, and critiques that have helped to train me as a researcher and to move forward with my research;

Vincenzo Romania for his availability and support;

Andrew Abbott, who welcomed me to the University of Chicago for three months, for the exchanges, suggestions, and reflections that stimulated and guided my work;

And many others, in strict alphabetical order: Valerio Belotti, Carla Bertolo, Matteo Bortolini, Francesca Campomori, Alberta Contarello, Salvatore La Mendola, Devi Sacchetto, and Luca Trappolin, because our exchanges, sometimes rapid and in other cases more in-depth, allowed me to advance as a researcher and as a person;

Christine H. Morton, the premier doula researcher in the U.S.A., who welcomed my research project from the first moment I contacted her, and shared materials, reflections, and encouragement;

Sharon Hicks-Bartlett of the University of Chicago, who allowed me to take her course despite not having the credentials to attend it, accompanying me in my studies with generosity, and urging me to write;

Catherine Mardikes, bibliographer in the library of the University of Chicago, who accompanied and supported me with tenacity and dedication in the investigation of the Greek origin of the word "doula," and then welcomed me into her home on Thanksgiving Day.

A debt of gratitude is also owed to Brenda Benaglia, Martin Cecchi, Francesco Della Puppa, Eriselda Shkopi, Giulia Storato, Angela Maria Toffanin, and Francesca Alice Vianello, for their presence, feedback, support, and friendship.

A special thanks to Robbie Davis-Floyd, the lead editor of the Routledge series *Social Science Perspectives on Childbirth and Reproduction*, in which this book found its home, for her patient, precise, and constructive editorial support during the writing of this book.

I'm really thankful to Anna Villa, who gave me a much-needed physical space to write this book and who shared with me reflections and difficulties.

Finally, I'm deeply grateful to my family and friends:

To my husband Carlo, who nourishes me with his love, patience, and unwavering support, and to my daughter Adele, an engine of creativity who made me discover an everlasting love that grows day by day.

I also thank my parents Anna Maria and Giovanni, and my sister Marika, whose love and encouragement are ever present.

And a deep thanks to my best friends Marina, Sara, and Serena for always being there to share laughs, difficulties, and desires.

Introduction

What are doulas?

In most countries, the doula is a professional who offers practical, emotional, and informational support to the mother and family during pregnancy, birth, and the postpartum period. Yet in Italy, doulas support childbearers from pregnancy throughout the first year of the baby's life. Additionally, the majority of Italian doulas support women experiencing miscarriages, abortions, stillbirths, and assisted conceptions. Doulas are nonmedical professionals, but literature highlights that the presence of a doula supports physiological birth and healthier outcomes for mothers and babies (Hodnett et al. 2013).

Yet in truth, doulas are much more than the above description:

> Doulas are professionals who take care of mothers and mothers-to-be, while empowering those mothers and families.
> Doulas embody innovative ways of caring, offering flexible and individualized support.
> Doulas merge different systems of knowledge to respond to mothers and families' needs.
> Doulas trust in mothers and in their intuitive knowledge.
> Doulas do not tell childbearers what to do; rather they offer information to help them make their own choices.
> Doulas support mothers and families *without judging*, regardless of the choices related to pregnancy, childbirth, and the postpartum that mothers and families make.
> Doulas use a gentle and cozy approach; they hold a safe and comfortable space for mothers and families.

The first author to introduce the word "doula" was anthropologist Dana Raphael in 1966. In her PhD research about breastfeeding in different cultures and in some animal groups, Raphael identified the common denominator for success in breastfeeding, which consists of some degree of help for the new mother from some specific individual, for a precise period after childbirth.

DOI: 10.4324/9781003165934-1

Raphael (1969) decided to use the word doula to name the profile that fulfils these functions. The term doula is of Ancient Greek derivation: δούλη (in Modern Greek δούλα) is a female noun indicating a slave or servant. The term proposed by Raphael was later embraced by US pediatricians and researchers Marshall Klaus and John Kennell (Klaus et al. 1986, 1993; Kennell et al. 1991), who expanded its meaning to define a doula as a woman experienced in childbirth assistance who provides information and continuous physical and emotional support before, during, and immediately after the delivery, thereby enshrining the current definition of the term "doula."

From time to time, women used to support mothers-to-be and new mothers, as my 100-year-old grandmother has always told me: after each of her four births, she spent 40 days lying and resting in the bed, while her mother-in-law dealt with all chores. Nevertheless, the consequences of the social, cultural, and economic changes that occurred in the 20th century often impeded family and friend networks from supporting the pregnant or "newborn" mother, while simultaneously the process of medicalization of the procreative event and the transfer of childbirth to the hospital took place. The biomedicalization of birth, with its lack of empathy and compassion, and often the lack of a supportive network, generates in expectant and laboring women and in new mothers the need for emotional and practical support that used to be filled by her network of family and friends—and now can be fulfilled by the doula.

The doula emerged in the U.S.A. between the 1980s and 1990s, in Europe by the early 2000s, and nowadays they are widespread worldwide. This book focuses on the fairly recent development of doulas in Italy, where the first doula training took place in 2007. Nowadays, several associations offer trainings, and Italian doulas are growing in numbers, despite the opposition to their emergence by the National Federation of Midwives. This scenario is challenging and fraught, since some midwives do not agree with their national federation and wish to support and collaborate with doulas.

A personal note

The first time I heard the word doula was in 2012. Intrigued by the description of this figure, I began to investigate and discovered that in a few months, a doula training would begin in my area. I looked at the program, reflected about it, and talked to the trainer. I didn't know anything about motherhood, I was not a mother, I had never met this theme in my studies, but I was nevertheless attracted, and decided to enroll. I started my doula training in October 2012, and a few days later, I also passed the entrance exam for my PhD, for which my education started in January 2013. The first months of 2013 were full of academic coursework, but in the remaining time, my curiosity increased, and I began to carry out research on doulas worldwide. I discovered the existence of studies that investigated the medical benefits of doulas working with pregnant and delivering mothers, which include reduction in the use of drugs, reduction in the time of labor, and reduction in the number of caesarean births (Sosa et al. 1980; Campero et al. 1998; Hodnett 1999; Kayne et al. 2001; Campbell et al. 2006; Berg and Terstad 2006; Akhavan and Lundgren 2012; Hodnett et al. 2013; Bohren et al. 2019). I also discovered a body of research that investigated the doula from sociological, anthropological, and philosophical points of view (Morton 2002; Gilliland 2002; Meltzer 2004; Henrion 2008; He 2011; Basile 2012; Morton and Clift 2014; Henley 2015; Castañeda and Searcy 2015). Most of these social scientists' work was developed in the U.S.A., and this attracted my attention. At that very moment, I decided that the time was ripe to devote my PhD dissertation research to studying Italian doulas; in the meantime, in June 2013, I completed my training and "officially" became a doula, slowly starting to take on clients. I thus also became the first Italian sociologist to both be a doula and to carry out research on doulas as they were emerging in my country. Some years later, in 2019, I got pregnant and was cuddled and coddled by two doulas and two midwives. The birth of my daughter was accompanied for me by a surge of creativity that pushed me to write this book, which is based on my dissertation research.

A methodological note

From the very beginning, the concern that most characterized my work has been related to my standpoint. I knew that being a doula would facilitate my access to my field of study and my understanding of the doula profile, yet at the same time, I was worried about being too involved and how I might take what originally seemed to me to be a necessary critical distance from my research. A sociological classic gave me the key to resolving this concern. Wright Mills, in his appendix to "The Sociological Imagination," (1959) wrote that the most admirable thinkers within the scholarly community do not split their work from their lives. They seem to take both too seriously to allow such dissociation, and they want to use each for the enrichment of the other. This key gave me a great deal of encouragement!

Reflecting on my standpoint, I envisioned the limits in the "insider vs. outsider" dichotomy (Merton 1972; Adler and Adler 1987; Kanuha 2000; Merriam et al. 2001; Asselin 2003) and felt the need to explore what Corbin Dwyer and Buckle (2009) have defined as the "space in-between." In this space, in-between these two poles, I carried out my research. Belonging to the group of doulas resulted in a fluid, procedural, and relational standpoint that needed to be defined from time to time, from moment to moment, and from person to person. Certain elements influenced this process. First of all, I was practicing as a doula and had become a member of one of the main Italian doula associations. This membership and all that it entails may have influenced my choice of interlocutors and the interlocutors themselves, many of whom were members of associations different from mine. In those cases, I anchored myself in my role as researcher, and this worked to avoid creating frictions during the interviews I carried out and enabled me to deepen my research into the topics regarding doulas that most interested me. A second element that affected my fluid movement in the "space in-between" was my personal knowledge of some of the interlocutors. This allowed me to easily delve into my research field. Nevertheless, being an insider did not mean having free access to all doula events (Riessman 1987; Beoku-Betts 1994).

A further element that urged reflection was constituted by the expectations of some doulas in relation to my research; as Dina put it, "I think a PhD from Dr. Pasian [laughs] will be very important. I think that even research can be a good way for the profession to grow. People who do research can give officiality to the profession." The responsibilities to address the subject of doulas in Italy via sociological research for the first time and to not disappoint the expectations of those doulas who for years have been looking for a form of institutional recognition, required long moments of reflection and a constant questioning of my interpretations. In addition, I asked myself: "Why not include your emotions in your research?"

I felt a sort of fear about including my emotions, probably due to the stereotype that still characterizes Euro-American intellectual circles and is based on the Cartesian mind-body dichotomy, which holds that emotions disturb knowledge, are pre-social, and must be controlled and regulated by rationality (Sclavi 2003). As highlighted by La Mendola (2009), the "reflexive turning point" (Melucci 1998) has had the great merit of opening important interpretive perspectives recognizing the involvement of the researcher in generating the interactions and in evidencing the connection of the process of reflexivity with research practices. However, this type of reflexivity still remains too rational and too anchored to the left hemisphere of the brain. In fact, theories of "reflexivity" do not attend adequately to emotions (Holmes 2010); rather they involve mental processes of self-reflection.

Wishing to take a more holistic approach, I decided to consider emotions as constitutive elements of the reflective/reflexive process. Emotions are essential elements for the start of the reflective process and for its feeding; it is not possible to separate reflexivity from emotion as disconnected elements; rather, they form a continuum. Therefore, I decided to adopt an "emotional reflexivity" approach (Holmes 2010, 2015; Burkitt 2012) in my work, by which I mean that embodied and relational process through which social actors become aware of their emotions and make them an integral part of their own reflective processes. The assumption underlying this approach is that all emotions are relational phenomena generated in the exchange and interactions in which we researchers are involved (Denzin 1984). The relational aspect is also decisive in the analysis and interpretation of the data, since the memory of the emotions felt during interviews or participant observation will inform the process of data analysis. Widening emotional repertoires are essential not only to enlarge the scenarios and possible interpretive frames in attempts to understand the complexity of society

(Sclavi 2003) but also to identify new methodological and epistemological frameworks.

In that process, I had to define the subject of my research among the many possibilities for it. I decided to start from the beginning of what seemed a fundamental incipient story that could give rise to many other developments. My choice, as previously noted, has been to focus on the profile of the doula in Italy, identifying her characteristics and peculiarities, and investigating the multiple ways in which doulas are emerging and entering the system of maternity care professions. Gathering representations of doulas and analyzing the meanings they attribute to their practices constituted the path I chose to grasp that ongoing process, as it allowed me to observe the dynamics and evolutions in their making. My choice was also influenced by my insider perspective and my preexisting knowledge about the most-discussed topics among doulas.

Starting from the development of the doula at the international level, this book describes and analyzes the origins, characteristics, and practices that distinguish doula work from that of other maternity care professionals, with the aim of outlining professional doula culture in Italy. The different types of doulas, according to the meanings they attribute to their work and to the conflicting and cooperative relationships with professional midwives, will allow us to understand the complexities and opportunities of an emerging profession. From the sociological tradition of the Chicago School (Hughes 1958), and in particular from the theorization developed by Andrew Abbott (1988), I adopted the concept of *professions* as a reference point. Professions are constituted by groups of individuals who gain and claim control of a specific area of work (Abbott 2010). The appearance of a "new" profession committed to gaining control of a certain area of work urges the "established professions" to evolve and reshape. Therefore, professions are interlinked in a perpetual movement of reciprocity that involves them in a process of *doing*, *redoing*, and *undoing*. For this reason, I considered it important to also collect professional midwives' representations of doulas, as midwives are the professional group with which Italian doulas interact the most. If, as Elias (2007) states, a profession is born to respond to new or unsatisfied needs but also to deficiencies, defects, or "bad adaptations" of preexisting institutions and professions, my study could not fail to consider the midwifery profession in Italy, most especially given the opposition that the National Federation of Midwives (Fnopo)—the organization within which all midwives must be registered—has always publicly expressed to the emergence of doulas— because the rise of doulas in Italy has highlighted, to their resentment and dismay, midwives' failures to fulfill the full range of childbearing women's needs for support.

The book is based on sociological research realized through literature review, interviews, and participant observation. My interviews with doulas and midwives were characterized by the same methodological approach, based on the ethno-sociological model proposed by Bertaux (1999) and the dialogue approach developed by La Mendola (2009). These interviews were accompanied by my ethnographic activities in doula trainings and social events. In these contexts, I took part in such activities as both a doula and a sociologist, and my diaries alternate in a fluid way among observational, methodological, theoretical, emotional notes (Corsaro 1985; Gobo 2001), and autoethnographic passages (Ellis 1995, Ellis et al. 2011).

Between 2014 and 2015, I conducted 32 interviews with doulas, 4 interviews with privileged actors (people who know the field well and can provide useful information about important facts related to the research topic), and 14 interviews with midwives. To interview doulas, I followed two parallel paths. On the one hand, I referred to the five associations that were offering trainings during the time period of my research—Mondo Doula, Mammadoula, Adi-Associazione Doule Italia, Progetto Primo Respiro, and 13 Doule. I contacted the members of these associations whom I knew personally, and in cases where I did not have personal knowledge, I contacted the association presidents, who mediated my contact with the doulas for the interviews. The condition that I placed as necessary before proceeding with the interviews was that the interlocutors had at least one year's experience working as doulas. The doulas interviewed form an extremely heterogeneous group in terms of age, training, and employment. A characteristic that they share concerns their areas of residence; they all live in regions of North and Central Italy; the presence of doulas in the Southern regions is scarce. The interlocutors range in age from 27 to 59 years. They have high to medium levels of education: 10 have obtained a high-school diploma, 20 have a Master's degree, and 2 have a PhD. Their educations are mostly concentrated in the humanities and social fields (psychology, sociology, education sciences, communication sciences, and political sciences); four have had an artistic training (Conservatory, Academy of Fine Arts, Photography and Theatre), and three were educated in the fields of pharmaceutical, physical, and chemical sciences. It is interesting to note that among the doulas interviewed, 17 had abandoned their previous occupation and devoted themselves exclusively to doula work, while 15 have maintained their previous activities alongside those of the doula.

Of the 14 midwives interviewed, 3 were hospital midwives, 3 were community-based midwives, 4 were freelance midwives, 1 was a midwife who works part-time in a hospital and part-time as freelance, 1 was a university professor of a midwifery course, who was also vice president of the National Federation of Midwives, and 1 was a newly graduated, as yet unemployed midwife. In this way, I covered all working areas in which midwives are involved. The midwife interlocutors range in age between 24 and 61 years. I got in touch with these midwives via emails or through personal contacts. My standpoint has generated many reflections and questions also with respect to my interviews with midwives. I did not want to hide the fact that I was a doula, but at the same time, I didn't want to compromise the development of the interview. It was clear to me that declaring my doula identity at the beginning of the meeting could influence the success of the interview, considering many midwives' opposition to doulas. So, I decided to introduce myself as a PhD candidate, and only at the end of the interview did I reveal that I am also a doula. At that point, a relationship had already been established between me and the midwife, the interview was officially over, and there was space for discussion. This space has proved interesting and fruitful. All data collected were fully transcribed, coded (Saldaña 2013), and analyzed through the software MAXQDA.

The structure of this book

I have organized this book into six chapters. Chapter 1 explores doulas worldwide. Starting from the first use of the word doula as a supporting figure, I trace the evolution of the term. I also investigate and reconstruct the evolution of the doula in the U.S.A. and Europe. Finally, I present a view of different research paths about doulas, and outline the specific declinations of the multiple ways of *doulaing*. Chapter 2 traces the development of doulas in Italy, reconstructing their paths—thanks to the voices of the first Italian doulas and professionals who influenced the cultural environment that encouraged the emergence of the doula. I narrate the origin stories used by Italian doulas to explain the historical background of the profile and the legislative framework that rules the doula profession in Italy. I conclude this chapter by describing the opposition to the emergence of doulas from the midwives' national federation and with some contextual data about birth in Italy.

In Chapter 3, I present a comparison between the Continental European and the Anglo-American traditions regarding the professions, which opens a number of reflections from the sociology of professions, from the feminist and philosophical literature, and from the health and reproduction sectors of sociology and anthropology, to affirm that the doula is a social care profession. As midwifery is the profession of midwives, and nurs*ing* is the profession of nurses, the profession of doulas in English can be named doulaing. This emergent profession is based on an innovative model of care through which doulas work to transform the cultural, technocratic approach to maternity care into a humanistic approach that encompasses relationship-based care and keeps the woman at the center of that care (Davis-Floyd 2001, 2018, 2022).

In Chapter 4, I analyze the programs of three trainings to become a doula in Italy, focusing on practical, physical, and emotional skills, on doulas' techniques and practices, and on some ritual and relational models that characterize doula trainings. The system of knowledge to which the doula refers is pluralistic and has a specific type of coherence that I label "patchwork"—as in a quilt of many pieces and colors that nevertheless has a coherent design. Doula practices give coherence to the pluralism of symbols and systems of knowledge to which the doulas refer and which they incorporate and practice as professionals. Chapter 5 focuses on the features characterizing doulas' work and the relations within the professional group. Doulas attribute different meanings to their work, allowing me to identify three ideological types of doulas: the "progressive doula," the "philanthropic doula," and the "individualistic doula." I also show that, despite these elements of internal differentiation, the adoption of a rhetoric of sisterhood and solidarity that embodies fundamental aspects of the doula profession overcomes differences and strengthens bonds that can ensure the ongoing development of doulas in Italy, whereas in other countries, doulas have not developed this kind of sisterhood and solidarity, but rather have split into factions with controversial relationships. Finally, Chapter 6 deals with the theme of interprofessional relations and focuses in particular on doulas' relationships with midwives. Starting with a reconstruction of midwives' professional history in Italy, this chapter delves into the opposition to the emergence of the doula by the representative bodies of professional midwives. I show that some midwives are willing to cooperate with doulas, recognizing the value of their support. This willingness evidences an ongoing process in which professional boundaries are in flux as midwives fight, or adapt to, the presence of the professional doula in Italian maternity care.

In sum, this book constitutes an in-depth exploration of Italian doulas. In it, I examine their relatively recent emergence and development; their professional status within the country; their ideologies and knowledge systems; the trainings and associations they have developed and the difference among these; and their interprofessional and often-problematic relationships with midwives. I also explore the relationships these doulas develop with the childbearers they attend, the multiple, year-long services they provide to those women, and the sociocultural and professional spaces they are creating for themselves as professionals serving women and as agents of change in Italian birth.

1 Doulas: From their origins to their present status

The origin of the word "doula"

As noted in Introduction to this volume, the first author to introduce the word "doula" was Dana Raphael in 1966. Raphael, an anthropologist and pupil of the famous anthropologist Margaret Mead, devoted her PhD research to the topic of breastfeeding in different cultures and in some animal groups. Raphael (1966) affirmed that her personal failure to breastfeed her first child stimulated her interest in studying varying experiences of motherhood, in order to understand what factors could influence breastfeeding success. Her work identified the common denominator for success in breastfeeding, which consists of some degree of help for the new mother, from some specific person, for a precise period after childbirth. Raphael discovered the presence in many cultures and animal species of such a support figure. She highlighted how this role was occasionally covered in the U.S.A. by a figure called "auntie"; however, she considered this term unsatisfactory for describing the systematic support to the new mother that she had observed in other cultures and in animal groups. Instead, she decided to identify the profile that fulfills these functions with the word doula (Raphael 1969).

Raphael noted that the term doula is of Ancient Greek derivation: δούλη (in Modern Greek δούλα), a female noun indicating a slave or servant. According to Raphael, in the 19th century, the negative meaning of the word disappeared and the term δούλια (doula) was used in an honorific sense and distinguished Greeks and Christians from Turks or "infidels." The word doula thus acquired an aura of respectability that was later lost again. At that time, in the 19th century in Greece, the term was used to denote a woman who assisted a new mother by supporting her in housework and with children. The doula could be a neighbor, a relative, or a friend who voluntarily supported the woman for a limited period of time (Raphael 1969).

Raphael does not include any bibliographical references in her writings in relation to the origin, the meaning, and the positive sense that the term doula might have acquired at the end of the 19th century. The sole information in

DOI: 10.4324/9781003165934-2

this regard was provided on the website of the Human Lactation Center,[1] which Raphael founded with Margaret Mead in 1975, where Raphael stated that a Greek woman, who had immigrated to the U.S.A. at the beginning of the 20th century, suggested the term doula and described her specific role.

In order to verify the reliability of the Raphael's statements about the positive meaning acquired by the word doula in the 19th century, I got in touch and started an intense correspondence with Maria Andreoulaki, Co-Founder and Coordinator of the Educational Committee for the Doula Certification program in Greece through the Greek Doula Association. Andreoulaki represented the Greek Doula Association during the European Doula Network (EDN) meeting, held in Portugal in 2014, giving a lecture entitled "Doula: from an ancient Greek word to a modern international reality." Andreoulaki, who conducted a great deal of research to understand the origin of the word doula, considers unlikely the positive 19th-century meaning attributed to the term by Raphael. Andreoulaki hypothesizes a possible misunderstanding between Raphael and the elderly Greek woman for two main reasons. First, Greek emigration at the end of the 19th century was characterized by poor, often illiterate people fleeing post-war crisis, civil war, and very poor living conditions, and consequently, according to Andreoulaki, the elderly woman's command of English could not have been sufficient to allow an accurate description of the doula profile. Second, Greeks were allegedly called "slaves" by Turks, and the word doula could indeed possibly have been a reassuring means to define themselves as Christians. Raphael decided, perhaps incorrectly, to rely on the story of the elderly woman. And considering the correspondence between the doula functions described by that woman and the activities carried out by the support figures present in the cultures and animal groups she investigated, Raphael (1973:172) chose to adopt the term doula to define "one or more individuals, often female, who give psychological and physical assistance to the newly-delivered mother."

The term proposed by Raphael was later embraced by influential researchers Marshall Klaus and John Kennell (as I will describe later on), who expanded its meaning to define a doula as a woman experienced in childbirth assistance who provides information and continuous physical and emotional support before, during, and immediately after the delivery, thus enshrining the current definition of the term doula. It is interesting to note that this word and its related profile were initially established in the U.S.A. and Europe and gradually spread worldwide. According to Andreoulaki, the only country in the world where the word is considered unacceptable and unusable is Greece, where the term maintains its negative connotation of servant or slave. However, during international meetings, Greek doulas adhere to the widespread use of word doula to represent themselves.

---

1 http://www.thehumanlactationcenter.com I consulted this website in 2017; by January 2021, it had disappeared.

The international development of the doula

The development of doulas in the U.S.A.

The doula emerged in the U.S.A. between the 1980s and 1990s in response to the changes in the medical and social contexts of birth that had been occurring (Morton and Clift 2014). From the 1930s to the present, the U.S.A. experienced a succession of controversial processes: the hospitalization and medicalization of childbirth have over time been countered with the birth of movements aimed at promoting women's health, patients' rights, the demedicalization of labor and birth, and the use of non-conventional medicines. A number of patients' rights organizations were set up to develop advocacy activities aimed at satisfying women's wishes related to medical practices involving their bodies. According to Davis-Floyd (2022), from an earlier focus on "natural childbirth" and "alternative birth," the adoption of a rights-based humanistic paradigm in the biomedical–hospital–technocratic context became the objective to be pursued (Davis-Floyd 2001, 2018; Earp et al. 2008).

In those same years, scientific evidence on the importance of the doula's role in childbirth was consolidated by the work of neonatologist Marshall Klaus and pediatrician John Kennell and their numerous studies (Klaus et al. 1986, 1993; Kennell et al. 1991). These two researchers, interested in investigating factors that inhibited or favored mother–child bonding, discovered the figure of the doula described by Raphael (1973) and decided to adopt it as an explanation of the results that emerged from their earliest studies. The incident that marked their introduction of the term took place in a hospital in Guatemala, when a medical student who was collaborating with these researchers and their team never left women alone during labor. Her role should have been to stay true to the purpose of the study—the goal of which was to investigate factors that inhibited or favored mother–baby bonding—but she accidentally remained continuously next to every woman in labor to whom she was assigned for this research project. This was interpreted as a mistake and the ten mothers she had supported were excluded from the study. However, it was later decided to examine the data of the ten women previously excluded, and it emerged that their labors had been unusually short and without complications, and in three of them, there had been a very rapid production of colostrum after childbirth (Klaus et al. 1993). This fortuitous event inaugurated a series of studies carried out in different contexts, which confirmed that the continuous presence of a support figure, called a doula, reduced the number of caesarean sections by 50%, the duration of labor by 25%, the use of pitocin to augment labor by 40%, the use of analgesics by 30%, the use of forceps by 40%, and the demand for epidural analgesia by 60% (ibid.). These convincing results provided a solid scientific foundation for the introduction of the doula into the labor room, thereby helping to create an entirely new profession in the U.S.A.

The first doula trainings in the U.S.A. ran between 1979 and 1980 in The Birth Place, a freestanding birth center founded in 1979 in Menlo Park, California. The trainings, taught by various people with differing skills and perspectives that included the integration of mind, body, and spirit, and dealt with political issues and the history of birthing, were organized twice a year and were not well structured. In 1983, one of the trained doulas, Rahima Baldwin, decided to found an organization called the Association of Childbirth Assistants, which in the following year became the National Association of Childbirth Assistants (NACA). NACA later evolved into the still-extant ALACE—the Association of Labor Assistants and Childbirth Educators.

During the 1980s, the doula profile began to spread in the country, to receive more attention among childbirth professionals, and to be the subject of publications. Since then, numerous doula organizations have been formed at local, national, and international levels. In 1992, the Doulas of North America (DONA) association was founded by neonatologist Marshall Klaus, pediatrician John Kennell, psychologist Phyllis Klaus (Marshall's wife), perinatal educator Penny Simkin, and doula Annie Kennedy. The first goal of these founders was to create an umbrella association able to define the training paths to becoming a doula in order to homogenize and certify the doula training programs that by then were spreading across country with considerable variations. Despite the fact that numerous doula associations decided not to merge into DONA, the association grew considerably as the number of members increased, and the use of the term doula started to be implemented and nationally recognized, thanks to specific trainings and advertising events, and to the personal reputations of the founders, who were and are still widely admired in the US birth activist community, which considers them to be "icons" and "culture heroes," both in life and in death (as Marshall and Phyllis Klaus and John Kennell are deceased). In 2004, having expanded its reach beyond the U.S.A., the association changed its name to DONA International. By September 2021, DONA International trained more than 12,000 doulas in 50 countries of the world and constitutes a reference point worldwide (www.dona.org).

Interestingly, an early controversy that arose between the founder of what later became ALACE, Rahima Baldwin, and the founders of DONA was whether or not doulas should be allowed to perform cervical checks to assess dilation at the laboring woman's request, usually to help her decide when to head to the hospital. According to Robbie Davis-Floyd (personal communication, September 2021), Rahima Baldwin was adamant that this should be part of doulas' skillset, while DONA was equally adamant that it should not. Since cervical checks carry dangers, such as infection, and are considered medical procedures that should only be performed by midwives or doctors, this controversy was ultimately resolved in favor of doulas not performing them. Thus, doulas learned many other methods of assessing labor progress, such as the sounds the mother makes, how she smells and acts, the kinds of breathing she does, and certain bodily changes. These skills matter most if the mother-to-be is laboring at home and needs to decide when to go to the hospital. Going too early, when she is still in latent labor, which can safely take hours or days to turn into active labor, can result in many interventions, a diagnosis of "failure to progress," and a cesarean birth. In the U.S.A., the doula's role has come to include going to the mother's home when labor begins, and helping her to decide when it's time to go to the hospital—should she be planning a hospital birth.

The development of doulas in Europe[2]

By the early 2000s, doulas had begun to proliferate in Europe, and new doula associations rapidly arose. In 2001, Doula UK was established in Great Britain, and in 2006, the association Doulas de France in France. In 2008, Doulas in Deutschland was born in Germany; in 2009, Eco-Mondo Doula[3] in Italy[4]; and in 2010, AED—Asociación Española de Doulas in Spain.

In 2005, a few European doulas started to share the need and the vision to establish quality standards for doula training and practice; reflections and discussions continued during a conference in Graz, Austria (2006), and at several birth-related conferences, including Midwifery Today conference in Bad Wildbad, Germany (2006 and 2008), and at a conference in Paris, France (2007). With the goal of creating a network of support and information among the various doula training providers and associations in Europe, this group of European doulas undertook a six-year path. In 2006, the association Doulas de France set up a Yahoo site with the idea of generating a focal point where doulas could network and included in their annual meeting Journées des Doulas, a workshop dedicated to European doulas. In 2007, the Doulas de France created The European Doula Guide, which included descriptions of a number of European doula organizations. This was the first insight into the real scale and breadth of the doula movement across Europe. In 2008, a group of German-speaking doula trainers took the first steps to create a framework for unity and equal standards among German-speaking doula associations and training organizations. They created a document shared with all the European doula associations they knew of, in order to collect and complete numbers, training standards, and information from all over Europe. This group of doulas set up the first EDN website and presented it

2 Many thanks to Regula Brunner, Valérie Dupin, and Sabine Lanfranchi (in alphabetical order of surname) as founding members of EDN, and to Mary Kalau as former EDN Office representative and EDN Newsletter editor, who contributed to the writing of this paragraph. In addition, many thanks to Debbie Mitchell and Maria Andreoulaki, from the EDN Office team. All of them generously and freely shared with me their time, notes, and memories.
3 The association Eco-Mondo Doula changed its statute and name in 2017; now its name is Mondo Doula.
4 This short list aims at giving an example of the diffusion of the profile and is not exhaustive.

during the Journées des Doulas de France in Paris in 2011. At this occasion, the EDN was officially founded. Participants in this meeting included doulas from the United Kingdom, the Netherlands, Hungary, France, Switzerland, and Germany.

The founders decided to schedule an annual gathering of doula representatives of the various training organizations and associations, hosted by a different member country each time. The aim was to exchange information and learn from each other, in order to gain a deeper understanding of challenges faced by birthing communities in each nation. The following meetings took place in Holland (2012); Switzerland (2013); Portugal (2014); the United Kingdom (2015); Spain (2016); Poland (2017); Austria (2018); the Czech Republic (2019); and online in 2020 due to the coronavirus pandemic. Since the first official gathering in 2012, these meetings have evolved to include all European doulas (not only organizational representatives), especially local doulas in the meeting host country. In 2013, EDN statutes were written, and during the 2015 EDN annual meeting, a Code of Ethics was created. Lawyer, charity trustee, and breastfeeding counselor Johanna Rhys-Davies assisted EDN representatives with creating a translatable document both in terms of language and of cultural sensitivity. It was crucial to give birth to a document that clearly stated the role of the doula, considering and including European countries' diversities in birth traditions, customs, and laws. Today, the EDN consists of 41 doula associations and training organizations that span 25 European nations, as well as many individual "friend" memberships that reach from the U.S.A. to Australia.

Research on doulas

The development of the doula profile was facilitated by the publication of several studies that have shown the benefits of the doula's presence. Medical and public health researchers were the first to investigate doula care. The results of these studies agree on the benefits of continuous support during labor and childbirth to reduce the duration, the use of drugs and analgesia, the rates of caesarean and operative vaginal births (with the use of forceps or a vacuum extractor—a small suction cup placed on the baby's head), and to create better bonding between mother and newborn (Sosa et al. 1980; Klaus and Kennell 1983; Klaus et al. 1986; Kennell et al. 1991; Hofmeyr et al. 1991; Simkin 1991; Klaus et al. 1993; Campero et al. 1998; Flamm et al. 1998; Goer 1995; Gordon et al. 1999). This branch of studies, which has continued to develop (Van Zandt et al. 2005; Campbell et al. 2006, 2007; McGrath and Kennell 2008; Mottl-Santiago et al. 2008; McComish and Visger 2009; Nommsen-Rivers et al. 2009; Hodnett et al. 2013; Chor et al. 2015; Kozhimannil et al. 2016), is characterized by an outcomes-oriented approach (Meltzer 2004). Some studies reveal that women who hire doulas develop increased self-esteem and feel more in control and emotionally supported (Rothman 1982; Simkin 1991; Zhang et al. 1996; Manning-Orenstein 1998; Hodnett 1999; Pascali-Bonaro and Kroeger 2004; Deitrick and Draves 2008).

Together with medical research, some social scientists and doulas decided to investigate the "doula phenomenon" (Morton 2002; Meltzer 2004; Gilliland 2010; Basile 2012; Morton and Clift 2014; Castañeda and Searcy 2015; Pasian 2015; Henley 2016; Benaglia 2018, 2020, 2022) by analyzing the practices and strategies that this profession adopts both to establish itself as a specific profile with its own expertise and to promote social change toward the humanization of birth. Currently, doula research is being implemented not only in Western countries but also in the Far and Middle East (Najafi et al. 2017; Chen and Lee 2020).

Doulas' services are becoming more and more specific as precise fields of intervention with determined targets are defined. Several studies have analyzed these processes, since the work of private doulas hired by the individual mother under the traditional model of one-on-one birth care is no longer the only way to practice the profession. Volunteer "community-based doulas," who work with young in age, low-income women and in general "serve communities that have been self-defined as underserved" (Breedlove 2005; Abramson et al. 2006; Gentry et al. 2010) represent one branch of this development. The major contributions made by community-based doulas of color during the COVID-19 pandemic in the U.S.A. are described by Oparah et al. (2021) and Rivera (2021), among others. Another branch is constituted by "prison doulas," who serve as a familiar presence from pregnancy to the postpartum for incarcerated mothers, supporting their mental health, well-being, and maternal empowerment (Schroeder and Bell 2005; Shlafer et al. 2015). "Indigenous doulas" constitute a new segment of this professional group; they work with women from Indigenous communities living in remote areas in Canada, Australia, and Greenland who are routinely evacuated to give birth alone and unsupported in urban hospitals (Kornelson and Grzybowski 2005; Varcoe et al. 2013; Ireland et al. 2019). Research on "radical doulas" in the U.S.A. (Basile 2015; Mahoney and Mitchell 2016) highlights the commitment of these doulas, who are trained within a reproductive justice framework, to support marginalized women and to resist their mistreatment by historically racist and sexist institutions. A debate among EDN members about radical doulas emphasized that it is not useful to separate doulas into "radical" and "non-radical," since their role is in itself always radical, inclusive, unbiased, non-judgmental, and human-rights-based. The situation is more complex in some countries, such as Russia, where supporting LGBTQ families can be interpreted as propaganda that supports homosexuality and is negatively sanctioned by law. Indeed, a Russian doula who stated her availability "to support LGBT families" on her Instagram page was forbidden to accompany childbearers in a local hospital. European doulas also discussed the idea of the "lay" doula, i.e. doulas who do not have "official" training. Lay doulas could constitute another branch of doulas, even though there is disagreement among European doulas on whether or not these women should even call themselves doulas, what services they should offer, and whether or not they should be admitted into professional doula organizations that generally require certification for admission.

A further development of the profile consists of "full-spectrum doulas," who offer support not only for labor and birth but also for all reproductive experiences, including abortion, adoption, miscarriage, and stillbirth (Basmajian 2014; Wilson et al. 2016). A further development of the doula profession that involves a different target population is "end-of-life doulas," who provide a diversity of non-medical support—social, emotional, practical, and spiritual—for people nearing death, including for those close to them (Krawczyk and Rush 2020; Rawlings et al. 2020).

Conclusion

In sum, in this chapter, I have described the origin of the word doula and its dissemination by anthropologist Dana Raphael. I traced the evolution of the term up to its current uses and described the multiple types of doulas currently in practice, exploring the development of doulas in the U.S.A. and Europe. Due to the lack of publications, I relied for my description of the development of the European Doula Network on the reports and the memories of the protagonists of the development of the European experience. I devoted the last section of the chapter to describing research on the effectiveness of doula care, including medical and social studies, as well as recent developments affecting the doula profession. In Chapter 2, I turn to the Italian case, describing the arising of the doula profession in Italy and its struggles with professional midwives in a perinatal context characterized by a high level of medicalization.

2 The emergence of doulas in Italy

The development of doulas in Italy

The figure of the doula emerged in Italy thanks to a cultural and social context that questioned the biomedical system, just as had happened in the U.S.A. and other countries. During the 20th century, the process of medicalization of the procreative event, from gestation to birth and beyond, and the transfer of childbirth to the hospital, established biomedicine as the exclusive sphere in charge of human reproduction. However, in the 1970s, the development of feminism, the popularity of women-empowering books such as *Our Bodies, Ourselves* of the Boston Women's Health Book Collective, and the creation of self-awareness groups prompted the calling into question of biomedical dominance. In this lively climate, during the 1980s, two organizations developed in Italy to promote—then and now—a vision of birth and motherhood that is based on the experiences and needs of childbearing women, and whose activities were fundamental for the subsequent development of the Italian doula.

In 1981, *Il Melograno*[1]—*Centro Informazione Maternità e Nascita* (Maternity and Birth Information Centre[2]) was established in Verona through the initiative of Tiziana Valpiana. This association had and has among its objectives: the promotion of a birth culture respectful of the physiologic rhythms of childbirth and of the intimacy and emotional needs of the couple and the child according to the indications of the World Health Organization; the promotion of the right to health and equal dignity of women and children; and the recognition of the social value of motherhood. To achieve these objectives, this organization aims to be a point of reference for women who wish to experience motherhood and childbirth as protagonists whose choices, individuality, and cultural preferences are respected.

---

1 The meaning of "melograno" is pomegranate, which is a recurring image in the Italian maternal literature.
2 My translation.

DOI: 10.4324/9781003165934-3

Tiziana explains:

> ... in our generation, for the first time, motherhood became a choice instead of an obligation ... on a personal level I decided to have a child ... I remember the first doctor's visit I did as if it were yesterday ... the doctor treated me like I had a cancer ... not a single word about the joy that I had of being pregnant. And leaving that clinic, I said ... "you won't have me!" On that day I thought, "but what do we need at this stage of life"? And I thought that we needed to talk to each other, to exclude all these worlds: psychologists, doctors etc., and to meet women to understand what it meant in a girl's life to choose to become a mother and then how to follow all these changes of the body first, of the relationship with the child from a point of view of reality, of women and of meaning, and so we decided to set up an association to allow women to share pregnancy and the postpartum period. We immediately thought that endo-gestation and exo-gestation can't be divided, are two aspects of the same adventure. So, we thought the most important need for women in those moments of their life could be to meet other women, share thoughts and insights.

The Melograno Centres have spread throughout the country and offer prepartum courses, assistance services across the perinatal period, parenting groups, meetings on specific topics, and breastfeeding support. In addition, a two-year "Master's in the art of mothering" course is still proposed to be aimed at those who want to take care of the accompaniment, support, and care of women and men in their becoming mothers and fathers.

The second organization to arise in the 1980s, precisely in 1985, was the MIPA—*Movimento Internazionale Parto Attivo* (International Movement for Active Birth[3]), founded by Piera Maghella in the city of Modena. The perinatal experience (pregnancy, childbirth, and postpartum) is considered by the MIPA to be a bio-psycho-social process that involves the body, relationships, and culture in which it takes place. The MIPA recognizes the centrality of the woman, the child, the couple with their skills and needs, and the right to have a "humanized" delivery in hospital or at home. The MIPA has organized trainings for women and couples in pregnancy, meetings for the protection and support of breastfeeding, gatherings of mothers and children, and also offers a training course for perinatal educators. The "perinatal educator" is defined by this organization as a social support person who holds meetings with mothers and couples in pregnancy and after birth, and proposes, informs, sensitizes, and facilitates meetings with health professionals.

Piera Maghella explains:

> I'm a perinatal educator ... My training took place in England, where I lived for ten years. I studied Educational Sciences with a Rogersian

3 My translation.

approach and then, in the meantime, I got pregnant for the first time and a world opened to me ... I realized the meaning of working with women. It is a very political act to support and help women to have the experience they want—it is a political act for me. First, I worked in two clinics and then in a hospital in England. I was paid by the National Health System, because the perinatal educator is a recognized figure ...

When I came back to Italy, I got scared. I already had two children born at home with the National Health System support in England—in that country, if a woman has a physiological pregnancy, she has the right to give birth at home and it is the National Health System that finds a midwife for you, if for example you live in a rural area. In Italy I got scared about the very low autonomy of the midwives ... that it is still so, the very little continuity of care that is still so, and the very little choice that women have on where and how to give birth. And then I got scared of the women' condition ... When I came back in '85, when a woman went to the hospital to give birth, she was bedridden. If one knows a little about physiology and how the body works, the last thing to do is tell a woman to stay bedridden, and then the cocktail of drugs they used in hospitals, and during the post-partum the excessive use of formula ... bottles in abundance, etc. ... Nowadays some things have improved, but what a fatigue! Back in Italy, I went to a public health center where I heard that the perinatal educator did not exist in Italy and there was no public placement for me, and from there I started the MIPA. Now, however, I also collaborate with the National Institute of Health (ISS) ... I was initially an unrecognized figure, but now they ask me to do trainings: I train the trainers of the Local Health Department ... now a space has opened up [for me].

Such experiences influenced the Italian cultural and social environment, as more and more attention was given to the needs of mothers and families. It was in this context that the term *doula* appeared in Italy. At the end of the 1990s, Massimo Canalicchio, an Umbrian father who worked as European projects planner, returned to Italy after living in the Netherlands, where his wife had delivered. He realized the considerable differences between the support that mothers received during pregnancy and after birth in the Netherlands and in Italy. So he decided to propose a project to the Umbria Region, the goal of which was the training of people to support new mothers. The Department of Health of the Umbria Region welcomed this proposal, which obtained the financial support of the Leonardo Da Vinci Program of the European Union in 1999. The title of the project financed was HOME—Home Obstetrical Mothercare Experience—and involved many Italian and international partners, including partners in Italy, Greece, Romania, and United Kingdom. This project's goal was to define the profile of a new professional figure able to assist mother and newborn at home and to provide the necessary training for both midwives and home assistants, so that both could have the tools and knowledge to manage pregnancy, childbirth, and postpartum at home. The initial idea was to call this new professional figure doula, but the Greek partners, during a project meeting held in Athens, strongly expressed their opposition because of the negative meaning of the term in the Greek language. The request of the Greek partners was accepted, after an intense debate, and it was decided to name the new professional profile "MA—Mother Assistant." The two training courses collected in a manual constituted the final product of the project, which obtained a positive evaluation from the European Union. In 2003, the province of Perugia, benefiting from funding from the European Social Fund, decided to implement the training model developed by the project HOME, activating a training course for the MA. Fifteen women attended the course, and in 2004, they founded the *AMA* (Mother Assistant Association).

Marina Toschi, gynecologist and head of the Equal Opportunities Center of the Umbria Region and coordinator of the project, stated:

> With this project I thought to find great enthusiasm from midwives, both because among the partners we had one midwife, and because from the 4000 questionnaires we collected emerged the need for mothers' support ... but no ... the Umbria Region and after it, the Province of Perugia, were denounced by the National Federation of Midwives, and brought to the Court, because this project and the course were [accused of being] against morality, women, science ... of course they lost; the Court, being competent in the matter, did not find any irregularities.

It is interesting to note that the opposition of the representative body of midwives was already evident in this pilot project. In the following sections, I will deepen the exploration of this topic. The training path to become a Mother Assistant was never repeated, but the need for people to support the new mother continued to be present, and within a short time, the first training paths for doulas were developed.

The first person in Italy to call herself a doula was Virginai Mereu, in 2000. She created the website www.doula.it. Virginia, graduated as Montessori children's community assistant, initially worked in a kindergarten and then focused on home support in labor and postpartum. Virginia uses different profiles to explain her profession: prenatal educator, mother's aide, child caregiver, and doula. Although each of these terms has specific characteristics, Virginia treats them as synonyms, since each bases its activity in the experience gained in her 40 years of work with new mothers. Even for Virginia, at the beginning of her career as a doula, there was a moment of tension with a midwife. In her interview, she stated that after four years of activity, she received an offensive email from a midwife accusing her of dealing with a sector in which she had no competence. So Virginia decided to rely on a lawyer, who responded to the accusations by defining her areas of competence, and from then on there were no other unpleasant episodes.

Seven years later, in 2007, the first Italian doula school was founded by Emanuela Geraci and Maria Grazia Biagini in Pisa. Emanuela's personal childbirth experience, when she was still a university student, was the trigger for this process. Emanuela said that, thanks to the support of her friends, all of whom were also university students, she was able to complete her studies and graduate in History. The support of her friends was fundamental in her experience, but she soon realized that few people deeply understood what it means to become a mother. After graduation, she decided to attend a counseling course, in which she acquired the tools to propose a training for childbirth as she would have wished for herself: full of fantasy, play, and creativity. In 2004, she began to work as a doula, after attending the courses of Childbirth International to learn to be a birth and postpartum doula. While at a party, she met Maria, a freelance midwife, who immediately proposed that they work together. As their collaboration was starting, Emanuela began to receive requests for information from women interested in the profile of the doula, so in 2007, the two friends and collaborators started the first doula training course in Italy. In 2009, they founded the Association Eco-Mondo Doula,[4] which offers yearly doula training courses and ongoing trainings for professional doulas, as well as a Summer School open to anyone interested in maternity-related topics. This association is part of the European Doula Network, has around 400 members, and has trained almost 900 doulas.

In 2006, Clara Scropetta, who had graduated in pharmaceutical chemistry, decided to quit her job at the pharmacy and change her lifestyle. She gave birth to her first child without any professional assistance, with the only support of her partner. This experience of what is generally termed "unassisted birth" developed her will to take birth back from the biomedical establishment. She travelled a great deal, deepening her understandings of the birthways of different cultures. When she returned to Italy, she began to support Michel Odent in the seminars he held in our country. After serving as a war doctor in Algeria and Guinea, Odent, a French physician, directed for 23 years, from 1962 to 1985, the services of surgery and obstetrics-maternity in the hospital of Pithiviers, in the department of Loiret in central France. During these years, Odent, who had originally been trained as a surgeon and knew little about birth (he was asked to head that department because he was the only doctor there), used his lack of official training in obstetrics as an advantage—he decided to learn from the Pithiviers midwives, who seemed to him to be doing a very good job. So, his initiation into obstetrics, unlike that of his colleagues, was an initiation into the midwifery model of care. Eventually he introduced the first *salle sauvage*, an environment similar to a home bedroom, a mediation between home birth and medicalized hospital delivery. These "salle sauvages" were quite womb-like, in that they

---

4 In 2017, the association changed its name in Mondo Doula. In the following pages, I will use the actual name.

were painted in dark, soothing colors and usually contained nothing but a comfortable bed on the floor. In them, women could move about freely and adopt any positions of their choice.

In 2007, Clara Scropetta, who has translated several of Odent's many books and is the author of the book *Accanto alla madre* (which I can translate as "being near to the mother") (2012), began to collaborate with the French doctor by proposing three-day residential trainings in Italy that culminated in the certification of *Paramanadoula*, which became recognized in the United Kingdom as well. During our interview, Clara wanted to clarify that she uses the word doula to define herself simply to facilitate the understanding of her work, while the definition that she feels most suitable to represent her is *custode della nascita* (which I can translate as "guardian of birth"). She feels that this term more completely describes her work, not only in reference to supporting women during pregnancy and childbirth but also in relation to the dissemination of a mother-sensitive culture around the country, which she implements through the organization of seminars, the presentation of books, and similar activities. Clara also offered to women and doulas an apprenticeship led by her: a program inspired by Jeannine Parvati Baker, an American midwife, yoga teacher, and natural birth activist (now deceased). This apprenticeship was to be carried out through personal or telephone meetings in which the apprentices ask for advice and guidance, while the trainer asks for questions or reflections and assigns tasks that can be carried out, or not, or can be transformed; Clara considers this "an apprenticeship in life." Clara is a charismatic figure, yet she is criticized by many doulas, as she agrees to attend women who wish to give birth without the support of any maternity care professional (midwife or ob). She considers it an issue related to the solidarity among women, in the awareness that she is not able to offer any obstetric support and with the pregnant woman's full assumption of responsibility. Her personal choice to support unassisted births clashes with the code of ethics of the main doula associations, which prohibit supporting unassisted births. Many doulas consider that this choice compromises their whole profession just as they are seeking to establish it *as* a profession. If a tragic event should occur, it would have negative repercussions on the entire professional group.

After the birth of the Doula School by the association Mondo Doula, other Italian doula trainings were created, such as those of the Cooperative *Piccoli Passi* of Sesto San Giovanni (Milan), the cooperative Pandora of Rome, and the Futures Association of Parma. The latter, in collaboration with the local health department, devised the Doula Project, which provided doula support to around 60 families. However, these trainings, which arose in response to calls for proposals and were funded publicly or by private foundations, did not prove to be sustainable and quickly disappeared.

In 2010, Laura Verdi founded Adi—*Associazione Doule Italia*—in Milan. Laura, who became a doula in 2002, has served as the president of this association since its foundation. In 2000, after some family troubles,

Laura decided to leave her job as commercial director in a multinational corporation and get closer to what she had always wanted to do: work in the maternal sphere. She enrolled in a two-year course taught by ANEP (National Association of Professional Educators) and began working as a prenatal educator, carrying out a three-year voluntary internship in a large hospital delivery ward in Milan. Laura's experiences in this delivery ward helped her to shape the profile of the doula and to understand how she as a doula could be most helpful during hospital labor and delivery. The Adi doula training program began in 2009; more than 50 doulas were trained in these Adi courses. Adi's ongoing activities consist of presentations, trainings, and seminars—some are public informational and cultural events, while others are reserved for members.

In 2011, Laura Verdi and Martina Bubola of the Cooperative Piccoli Passi began to collaborate, and, according to Italian law, transformed Adi from a minor association into an umbrella one for all the doula organizations spread throughout Italy, to facilitate the homogenization of training programs, with the goal of an institutional recognition of the doula. Later they changed the name of their training course to *Percorso per diventare doula di Laura Verdi* (Path to become Laura Verdi's doula). Laura chose this name as she wanted to underline that she was the creator of this original path.

During the 2010s, doulas began to be more active in their respective regions, to introduce themselves and their services into associations dealing with motherhood, or to found new organizations or projects: for example, the association *Mammadoula* was established in Rome; the association *Le Lune Allegre* (The Happy Moons) in Mestre; *Magicadoula* (Doula Magic) in Bologna; *Cerchi d'arcobaleno* (Rainbow Circles) in Padua; *Doula Mama* in Lombardy; and *L'abbraccio* (The Embrace) in the province of Turin.

In 2010, the association Mondo Doula was invited to carry out a training course in Bassano del Grappa (Vicenza-Veneto Region). When the course ended in March 2011, the 13 students who had participated decided to establish an association that would develop the activity of the doula in the Veneto region; thus, the association *13 Doule* was established. The activities of 13 Doule include the organization of events and public or private seminars aimed at members. The association also organized a (currently suspended) two-year training course with headquarters in Bassano del Grappa (Vicenza). Sixteen students were trained, and the presidency is entrusted to Chiara Pozzi Perteghella, pharmacist and doula.

In 2012, the first National Doula Conference, attended by 120 doulas, took place in Bologna. The aim of the meeting was to discuss and share the different experiences throughout the country and to lay the foundations for the construction of a solid network. The speakers represented the main national associations, and the topics covered included training, professional tools, language and some experiences, and good practices. The conference was a success; however, this has been the only national doula conference realized in the country.

In the same year as this conference, in Modena, a new training center for doulas was opened by the association *Circolo Primo Respiro* (First Breath Circle),[5] which had been active since 1999 with services aimed at women and families and focused on the periods of motherhood, fatherhood, breastfeeding, and early childhood and was introduced by Maria Chiara Purcaro, perinatal educator and doula. A new training path for doulas was implemented to promote the empowerment of women and the family. Maria Chiara considers access to doula support to be an investment in the health of women and, consequently, of the whole family.

In 2013, part of the board of Mondo Doula resigned and merged into the *Mammadoula* association, which was already operating in Rome. Mammadoula was transformed and became a national association with 51 members in 2014. This association, founded on the initiative of a group, not just a single person, considers the interactions, exchanges, and cohesion of its members to be fundamental. The activities they engage in include organizing not only events and seminars but also various types of projects aimed at social support to incarcerated women and to women living in foster homes. They also activated a training program.

The births of these various associations and the evolution of the doula profile garnered increasing interest on the parts of mothers, families, and public opinion. Major newspapers covered the topic of doulas, as well as numerous websites and blogs. In Milan and Turin, some private clinics and health centers decided to include doula services among the other services they offered. Although doulas in Italy have not yet been governmentally recognized, some public administrations have decided to sponsor, finance, or collaborate with projects and initiatives that promote or implement the doula. For example, the Addictions Department of the Local Health Unit in Trieste hired a doula to support a pregnant woman whom the service had in charge. Another project financed by the Province of Rome involved some doulas of the association Mammadoula. This project, *Adoulati mamma,* foresees providing doula support for pregnant women who live in situations of social hardship or who are inmates in Rebibbia Prison (Rome). This project attracted the attention of the Midwives Board in Rome, which wrote to the province to reiterate the absence of institutional recognition of the doula, to solicit a better investment of public money, and to request the suspension of activities. A commission was created with the aim of resolving the issue, all parties were involved, and the doulas won, ensuring the continuation of the project.

As previously noted, the interference of the National Federation of Midwives (Fnopo)[6] has accompanied doulas' activities since their very

5 In 2020, the association changed its name in Progetto Primo Respiro. In the following pages, I will use the current name.
6 The abbreviation of the National Federation of Midwives when the research was realized was FNCO. In this book, I will use Fnopo, as this is the actual name.

beginnings. In 2010, Laura Verdi of Adi received a warning from the Midwives' Board of Milan that generated the start of a technical table with the presence of their respective lawyers. The table aimed to define the respective areas of competence: Adi's statute was redrafted and their presentation brochure corrected. At the end of the process, the Interprovincial Board of Milan recognized doulas from Adi, and the agreement between the two organizations was also advertised on the site of the same board. However, the National Federation of Midwives has never approved of what the Milan board has achieved, considering this action dangerous for the entire midwifery profession. The intervention of the Federation in opposition to the activity of doulas took place through the press as well as through complaints and reports to the Public Prosecutor's Office, and for this reason, many training centers for doulas have been subjected to inspections by law enforcement agencies, which did not reveal any abuse of the midwifery profession.

It is important to understand that as doulas began to arrive on the scene in many countries, professional midwives began almost immediately to resent them, as the midwives considered the support of the laboring woman to be their exclusive purview. Yet it is also important to note here that these same midwives, or at least most of them, are part and parcel of the over-medicalization of birth and do not support laboring women in the ways that doulas do. Over time, in most countries where doulas have grown to large numbers, many midwives (and obstetricians) have come to appreciate the doula's role, as, especially in hospitals, one midwife is often caring for several laboring women at a time and thus can appreciate the value of continuous doula care. The midwife can leave the room knowing that the woman is still being nurtured. Such acceptance has obviously not yet occurred in Italy, where doulas are often not welcomed by hospital midwives. Moreover, in the majority of hospitals, there can be only one person to support the mother during birth; she has to choose between her partner and a doula.

Doula origin stories

When Italian doulas talk about the birth of the doula, they tell different narratives. One such story refers to mythology[7]; it identifies the first doula as a woman named Galanthis. Alcmene, the mistress of Zeus, is about to give birth to Heracles, and while the midwife is waiting, Galanthis, her handmaiden, struggles to understand what is not working, since for seven days and seven nights, Alcmene has been in pain trying to give birth to her son. Hera, the legitimate wife of Zeus, does not wish to allow the betrayal of her husband with Alcmene to result in the birth of Heracles; at stake is the right to reign over Thebes. And so to prevent the birth, Hera

7 The first time I heard this story was during the training course of the association "Mondo Doula" that I attended to become a doula in 2012.

engages Eileithyia, the goddess of childbirth. Galanthis enters and exits the room looking for a solution when she suddenly realizes that Eileithyia, to please Hera, is sitting on the lintel of the entrance door of Alcmena's birthing room with her legs, fingers, and arms crossed, preventing the birth with this spell. At this point, Galanthis devises a stratagem to allow the delivery to take place: she announces—lying—that her mistress had given birth and invites everyone to rejoice. Eileithyia, deeply astonished at the announcement, unties her limbs, thereby undoing the spell and allowing Alcmena to give birth to Heracles. After defeating the witchcraft of Eileithyia, Galanthis bursts into laughter, as she, a mortal, had succeeded in deceiving a goddess. Eileithyia, angered by falling into Galanthis's trap, decides to turn Galanthis into a weasel, which then became the symbol of doulas and midwives.

In "Metamorphoses," Ovid defines Galanthis as a *ministrarum*, generally translated as "one of the handmaidens," but Bettini (1998) points out that she was not a slave, since Ovid specifies that "she comes from the people" and that rules out the possibility of a having been a slave from birth. Galanthis is a person of modest condition compared to Alcmena, but she is free. Since she is not a slave and given the context, it is possible to affirm that Galanthis was an assistant "ready to execute commands" that the *obstetrix* or the most authoritative woman gave her. Bettini (1998) points out that Theban women knew this figure well and were grateful to her for the way she saved both Alcmena and Hercules. Also, Soranus of Ephesus, in his treatise *Gynaecology* (which was written around the 1st century AD and was translated into Latin in the 6th century by Muscio), reports that at the time of birth, there was not just one midwife, but a real team formed by the midwife and three assistants, named by him *huperétides*. In the Latin translations of the treatise, "assistants" bear the name *ministrae*, and *minister* is the technical term to designate the helper. Therefore, referring to mythology, the doulas anchor the existence of their profile in the support figure who *ministers* to women during childbirth and postpartum already present in ancient Greece.

The word *obstetrix* comes from the Latin word *obstare*, which I translate as "stand in front of"; it referred only to women. Its meaning explains exactly the position that the obstetrix had to assume during the birth. According to Gazzaniga (2014), the obstetrix was different from the *medicae* [doctor], since the latter had not only a practical but also a theoretical education, while the training of the obstetrix was likely to have been purely practical and experiential. This word, which has come down to us through history, is still in use in various forms in Italy and elsewhere. The Italian name for midwife is *ostetrica*, and the hospital ward where women deliver is called *ostetricia*, while *ginecologo/a* [gynaecologist] is the word for "obstetrician" (obs). In the Italian context, the midwife (ostetrica) is in charge of dealing with physiological pregnancy and birth, while the ob (ginecologo/a) is in charge of pathological pregnancy and birth. Nevertheless, the majority of newly pregnant Italian women choose an ob as their primary caregiver instead of a midwife, in this way reinforcing a medicalizing approach.

Another narrative about the birth of the doula refers to the history of women in Italy. For millennia, around the world gestation and childbirth were affairs of women—experiences lived within the circle of women and also events that drew meaning from a shared symbolic landscape. In Italy, a figure who played an important role in facilitating birth and the postpartum was the "levatrice"—also called by other synonyms such as *comare,* or *mammana*, depending on the regional area. She was a specialist in traditional folk medicine, essentially regarding women, and at the same time served as a magic-religious mediator in the complex rituals that marked the state of the pregnant woman and the newborn. In several European traditions, the role of psychological and symbolic support for the pregnant woman was predominantly compared to the "technical" role of the childbirth attendant (Giacomini 1992). The art of the Italian matron did not include nor foresee the use of "obstetric" instruments. Giacomini also pointed out that the presence of a group of women around the pregnant woman is evident in all the religious iconography in the different Nativities. However, between the 14th and 16th centuries, throughout Europe, the marginalization and denigration of women that accompanied the Renaissance and the exploitation of nature that promoted the transition to the modern era began to develop (Merchant 1988). The support of the matrons/midwives/doulas was progressively devalued, and around the middle of the 19th century, medical hegemony in the reproductive field began to be established. Today's Italian doulas, emphasizing the fact that women have always supported other women at the time of childbirth, and accusing the biomedical profession of removing this wisdom from women, express the ambition to, in a postmodern way, bring back some elements of a past in which women, their activities, and their ways of understanding themselves and their experience predominated during labor and birth and produced a specific kind of knowledge about how best to facilitate the birthing process (Pomata 1979; Davis-Floyd et al. 2018).

My final doula origin story refers to the work of Klaus and Kennell described in the preceding chapter, which, to recap, showed that the continuous support of a doula during labor and childbirth results in much more optimal outcomes: shorter duration of labor, lower rates of operative births (cesarean section, vacuum extraction, or forceps), less use of drugs, and also a heightened attention and awareness on the part of the mother immediately after birth (they caress, speak to, and smile at their newborns more than those who give birth without doula support). All these together have come to be called the *doula effect.* And the works of Kennell, Klaus, and others have shown that this doula effect only holds if the doula is *continuously* present with the laboring woman.

Following these initial studies, other randomized controlled trials (RCTs) were conducted worldwide confirming these results (see Hodnett et al. 2013). The effectiveness of doula support has therefore obtained, through these definitive studies, the validation professionals use to legitimize themselves. It is interesting, and paradoxical, that doulas anchor their history and legitimacy to medical-scientific knowledge obtained in RCTs but subsequently work to question, and occasionally counter, the same type of medical-scientific knowledge when it conflicts with their own knowledge about how to facilitate normal physiologic births and to support women in their emotional and psychological responses to their labor and birth experiences. It is also important to note that the doula research of Klaus, Kennell, and many others took decades to be accepted as legitimate in contexts such as the U.S.A, where doulas are still struggling today to be defined as "essential personnel" (Oparah et al. 2021; Rivera 2021). For example, during the coronavirus pandemic, hospitals that had formerly welcomed doulas immediately prohibited them from attending births because they were regarded as "non-essential" (Davis-Floyd et al. 2020).

Regulating doulas

In Italy, the system of professions is based on a legal framework of corporate institutionalization, which itself is based on institutionalized forms of control and social closure of access to professions (Maestripieri 2013). However, the economic difficulties that have affected Italy in recent years have pushed the issuing from the government of innovative regulatory solutions in favor of a more marked expansion of the free market. The set of deregulating measures implemented has resulted in a form of compromise between the need to ensure competition and the need to preserve constitutionally relevant assets and rights.

However, a review of the regulated professions has protected the constitutional principle that establishes that professions concerning the safety of citizens and the protection of the environment may be exercised only by those who have followed a specific course of study, have been qualified by a state examination, and are entrusted with the task of ensuring the quality of service through the rules of access to the profession and recurrent certification of its members. Yet, also in recent years, Italy has seen the development of numerous professions without specific legislative recognition and that have frequently created autonomous private professional associations. Such professions, which include for example educators, designers, photographers, and geophysicists, interest mainly the services sector and are defined unregulated. The role of such unregulated professions appears strategic in the Italian economic-productive system: the supply of qualified services to the enterprises involved increases competition and has positive implications in terms of innovation, while personal services and those in other fields (art, culture, education, and computer science) are inserted into areas in which the State does not always succeed in intervening effectively and efficiently

(Viciani 2015). The statute of unregulated professions (Law no. 4 of 14 January 2013 and art. 1, paragraph 2) reads:

> For the purposes of this law, 'unregulated profession', hereinafter referred to as 'profession', means economic activity, also organized, aimed at the provision of services or works in favor of third parties, usually and mainly exercised by intellectual work, or in any case with the help of this. (My translation)

This law introduced the principle of the free exercise of a profession based on autonomy, competence, and intellectual and technical independence and also recognizes that the professional activity can be carried out individually, within an association or corporation, or in the form of worker employment. Professionals can set up unregulated professional associations with the aim of enhancing the skills of members, spreading among them respect for ethical rules, and promoting user choice and protection, while respecting the rules of competition. A list of professional associations claiming to possess the characteristics required by the new law has been published on the website of the Ministry of Economic Development.[8] Law 4 of 2013 is the legal framework that legitimizes the work of the doula.

The Italian doula associations, understanding the importance of obtaining a form of legitimacy and institutional recognition, have taken some actions to pursue these goals, but these efforts have revealed a lack of coordination and cohesion among the organizations involved. In an attempt to harmonize the various doula associations present in Italy, and parallel to the institutional recognition efforts undertaken by some of them, a National Doula Coordination was begun. This Coordination was made up of representatives of the associations that offered a training course: Mondo Doula, Adi, Mammadoula, 13 Doule, and Progetto Primo Respiro. The Coordination's aim was to offer a space for reflection, to homogenize trainings, form a scientific committee to organize a second national doula convention, and create a common ethical charter for all the Italian doula members of the associations involved. The meetings of the Coordination group took place on 9 and 10 November 2013 and on 24 and 25 May 2014 in Bassano del Grappa (Vicenza). From the minutes of the second meeting, it was clear that three doula organizations had agreed to adhere to the homogenization/standardization of the training programs: Adi, Mammadoula, and 13 Doule. These minutes also showed that representatives from Mondo Doula did not provide feedback about the possibility of standardizing training programs, while Progetto Primo Respiro, although interested in following the work, did not attend the meetings. Adi, Mammadoula, and 13 Doule expressed some

8 The list is available on the web page of the Ministry of Economic Development, www.mise.gov.it/index.php/it/component/content/article?id=2027474:professioni-non-organizzate-in-ordini-o-collegi-elenco-delle-associazioni-professionali.

perplexities and asked questions about possible collaboration with Mondo Doula. The representative of Mondo Doula decided not to respond to the issues raised but to refer the questioners to a written communication. Mondo Doula responded to the points raised during the Coordination through an email of June 2014, which simultaneously communicated their decision to leave the Coordination. No other Coordination meetings have taken place since then; the process simply stopped. According to the former Mondo Doula Association's president, it was not possible to continue a reflection and co-construction path, because during the coordination meetings, the climate deteriorated and a spirit of real collaboration was lacking. However, these tensions seem confined to the executive board levels, without affecting the majority of doulas.

Midwives' opposition to doulas

As previously noted, the Italian National Federation of Midwives (Fnopo) has carried out an intense opposition to the figure of the doula. In several documents, the Fnopo tried to address the "problem" doula and/or other figures such as the mother assistant and the prenatal educator who, in the opinion of the Fnopo, are engaged in activities that are inextricably linked to the practice of midwives. In 1999, the Fnopo intervened legally for the first time, involving the Ministry of Health in reference to the training for prenatal educator, while in 2001, Fnopo lodged a complaint regarding doulas with the Public Prosecutor of Rome.

In the same year, the Fnopo consulted the Ministry in relation to the Project HOME, and in 2003, when the Umbria Region started the training implementing this Project's results, sent a notice to desist to the Ministry of Health, the Department of Health of the Umbria Region, and to the Court of Auditors and the Public Prosecutor's Office, asking "to remove all obstacles to the exercise of the profession of midwife and to inhibit any initiative detrimental to the dignity and professional autonomy of the midwife." Several times the Fnopo reiterated to the Ministry of Health reports concerning the activities of doulas in the Italian regions, and the Ministry replied, confirming that "such figures do not fall within the category of professions in the health area." Indeed, doulas are not healthcare professionals, as their role concerns the social and emotional sphere. In 2010, numerous midwives' city boards (Florence, Pisa, Turin, Milan, Venice, Udine/Pordenone, Varese, and Parma) reported the spread of the doula in their regions, the presence of more and more training courses, the inclusion of the doula in some health facilities in northern Italy, and in some cases required police investigations during doula trainings. In addition, the Fnopo verified the involvement of some midwives in doula trainings and in particular demanded that the National Federation Board working in the city of Pisa take action against one midwife, Maria Grazia Biagini, who was working in that area.

Maria Grazia Biagini, a freelance midwife who attended home births, founded with Emanuela Geraci the first Italian doula school in 2007, and together they trained doulas. During our interview, Maria told me that she had dedicated more than a year to creating the training program, because it was essential to think about the role of the doula in all its details. The aim was to provide the students in this doula school with the necessary tools to support childbearing women throughout the perinatal period via providing information and direct hands-on physical and emotional support. The program did not include any midwifery content. Biagini's doula trainings attracted the attention of her city Midwives' Board, which summoned her and instructed her to stop her trainings. Nevertheless, Biagini continued teaching at the doula school until in 2012, when the Board decided to sanction her with a disciplinary measure that obliged her to stop her activities for six months. The Board stated that the doula profession is not recognized by the Italian State and that Maria Grazia Biagini:

> takes part in the training of figures who may cause harm to the health of the woman and child, as well as to the family, since they are engaged in a profession not defined by Italian law and which abusively reproduces purely midwives' contents, thus creating confusion among users. The competence and professionalism of the midwife Biagini is not in question ... but the ideologically-based use of that expertise and midwife's knowledge [is]. (My translation)

Biagini decided to challenge her suspension by resorting to the Central Commission for Health Professionals, a body set up by the Ministry of Health and competent to resolve these types of issues. On 28 April 2014, the Commission confirmed the disciplinary measure that suspended the exercise of her profession for six months. From this moment, Maria Grazia Biagini no longer taught at her doula school and left the Mondo Doula Association. Maria's suspension was perceived as an injustice by Italian doulas, and numerous initiatives were implemented to express solidarity and support. A website was created; articles were published in magazines, websites, and blogs; crowdfunding was activated to support the midwife who could not work for six months; a letter was sent to the Ministry, one to the Federation, and European doulas of the European Doula Network also offered support. On the one hand, this activation of the Italian doulas was based on the fact that many had taken Biagini's trainings; thus, they could confirm the absence of medical equipment and midwifery content in her teachings. On the other hand, her supporters considered Biagini to be the victim of a corporatist system that obliged the founder of a school to leave it because she did not comply with hierarchically imposed dictates. Even many midwives dissociated themselves from the decision taken by the Central Commission.

Biagini, who associated her experience with similar episodes in history: "as if science were not covered with such experiences ... Should I quote Galileo?" acknowledged the shortsightedness of the decision: "The doulas will go on without me." Indeed, the doulas did go on without her and the schools continued to develop. These events strengthened the cohesion among Italian doulas who, via their networks and social media, began to collaborate intensively, regardless of any association membership. Thanks to this new spirit of collaboration, in a very short time, these doulas produced materials and initiatives. The same cannot be said for midwives. The decision regarding the suspension put many professional midwives in disagreement, generating discontent over the mismanagement of Biagini's case and fueling with yet another element the preexisting split among Italian midwives, which I will further discuss in Chapter 6.

Giving birth in Italy

The birth event is garnering more and more attention in Italy, both from women, who are increasing their awareness around birth, and by health policies that started to encourage physiologic delivery and improve the conditions in which birth takes place. Despite this attention, birth is still strongly medicalized, with a high use of cesarean section that disregards the recommendations for an appropriate and conscious choice of this surgery, present in the guidelines issued by WHO and the Italian Ministry of Health. Even during labor and spontaneous/vaginal childbirth, health professionals implement interventive practices that are rarely evidence-based.

According to data published by the Italian National Institute of Statistics[9] and the Ministry of Health,[10] and confirming the trends of previous years, in 2018, 62.83% of women delivered vaginally, while 32.32% were delivered by cesarean. The use of cesareans is widespread in a very heterogeneous way in the country, with higher rates in the south of Italy.

In 2014, WHO conducted a systematic review of the studies available in the literature, with the aim of identifying, critically assessing, and synthesizing the results of those studies that analyzed the associations between cesarean sections and maternal, perinatal, and infant outcomes (Betran et al. 2015). At the same time, WHO conducted a worldwide study to define the association between cesarean section and maternal and neonatal mortality (Ye et al. 2015). Based on these systematic reviews, WHO estimated that a rate of cesarean sections of up to 10%–15% at population level is associated with a reduction in maternal-neonatal and infant mortality. Above this percentage, cesareans are no longer associated with a reduction in mortality. The Italian average exceeds more than double the percentage indicated by WHO

9 www.istat.it/it/files//2018/03/La-salute-riproduttiva-della-donna.pdf.
10 www.salute.gov.it/imgs/C_17_pubblicazioni_3034_allegato.pdf.

and places Italy as having one of the highest cesarean section rates in the European Union (OECD 2019).

The birth defined as "vaginal" or "spontaneous" is not also "natural"—that is, without any medical intervention. On the contrary, medical intervention during labor and childbirth is frequent and takes the form of procedures that are often not evidence-based (see Davis-Floyd 2022). In 1985, WHO issued a document with recommendations for appropriate care during pregnancy, labor, and childbirth, as well as a practical guide in 1996 (WHO 1996), where it is expressly recommended to restrict certain practices to only specific cases of need. These practices include artificial rupture of membranes, which should usually be done only at an advanced stage of labor; electronic fetal monitoring to be performed only in particular situations; the systematic use of episiotomy, which is to be avoided because there is no scientific evidence showing effectiveness in reducing postpartum problems such as perineal lacerations and incontinence; and the routine administration of medications during labor, also to be avoided except in specific cases. A study implemented by the National Institute of Statistics in 2013 showed that the overall level of medical intervention in Italy is high: 72.7% of women with a vaginal delivery reported at least one medical intervention. Women reported rupture of membranes (amniotomy) in 32.1% of cases; the episiotomy rate was a shocking 34.6%; continuous fetal heart rate monitoring was used in 45.2% of cases; pressure on the abdomen in the ejective phase (including the harmful Kristeller maneuver) in 22.1%. Artificial oxytocin was administered to 22.3% of laboring women, but 14.2% reported not knowing whether or not it was injected. The use of forceps or vacuum extraction was 4.3%; this rate diminished as cesarean rates increased. These data confirm an excessive medicalization of childbirth in Italy that is unjustifiable by clinical necessity, as emphasized in the international and national guidelines for the biomedical treatment of birth. These Italian statistics are quite similar to those of many other countries, including the U.S. (except for episiotomies, which are now rarely performed in that country), showing the international over-medicalization of birth and the hegemony of what Davis-Floyd (2001, 2022) has called "the technocratic model of birth."

Considering place of birth, data collected in 2018 (Istat) show that, at the national level, 89.4% of Italian births took place in public hospitals, 10.5% in private clinics, and only 0.08% elsewhere (home or maternity home/birth center). In private clinics, 47.6% of the births are by cesarean, compared to 30.5% in public hospitals. Cesarean section is more frequent in women with Italian citizenship (33.7%) than in women from other countries (27.0%). 92.7% of births are supported by a partner, a family member (5.8%) or another trusted person, who may be a doula (1.5%); generally no support persons are allowed during cesarean births.

A positive note emerged from the National Institute of Statistics concerning breastfeeding. The WHO/UNICEF Joint Declaration (1989) underlined the importance of breastfeeding for the health of mother and child and set out the ten Steps of the Baby-friendly Hospital Initiative to promote, protect, and support breastfeeding. In particular, WHO recommends exclusive breastfeeding up to six months, and breastfeeding combined with other foods for as long as the mother and the child desire. In 2013, 85.5% of women in Italy breastfed in the five years before the survey, indicating a growth in the breastfeeding rate since 2005, when that rate was 81.1%. In addition, the average length of breastfeeding increased from 6.2 months in 2000 to 8.3 months in 2013.

Conclusion

In this chapter, I have explored the development of doulas in Italy, reconstructing their path thanks to the voices of the first Italian doulas, founders of doulas trainings, and professionals who influenced the cultural environment that encourages the emergence of the doula. I then described the narratives, or "origin stories," used by doulas to explain the historical background of the profile, and the legislative framework that rules the doula profession in Italy. My descriptions of the opposition to the emergence of doulas on the part of the midwives' national federation and this body's persecution of Maria Grazia Biagini had the goal of describing the complicated contexts in which Italian doulas work. I concluded this chapter by providing some data about birth in Italy to highlight the remarkable level of medicalization still present in this country, thereby revealing the need for doulas' efforts to humanize the birth experience.

3   Keys for studying the doula profession

To study how a profession emerges in a precise context and historical moment, it is necessary to pay attention to a multiplicity of elements, capturing the reflections offered by theories that frame different phenomena according to differing points of observation. As I have shown in previous chapters, the doula profile has started to develop in Italy in recent years, merging various knowledge systems and operationalizing a definition of skills with the aim of defining its cognitive corpus, or body of knowledge. Since a profession is always inserted into a specific historical and relational context, it is necessary to widen the gaze to the adjacent fields, especially to the biomedical field, in order to investigate how the definitions of boundaries between professions take shape. As described during interviews, the doula carries out typical care professions tasks; to understand these requires us to reflect on the process of care. The meaning that the protagonists of the profession attribute to that profession is intimately connected to the construction of the professional style that doulas incorporate and that, despite some differentiations and specificities, explicitly exhibits features of social care professions in general.

The concept of a profession in the Continental Europe and Anglo-American traditions

The concept of a profession has been the subject of intense debates and reflections (Carr-Saunders and Wilson 1933; Greenwood 1957; Millerson 1964; Wilensky 1964; Etzioni 1970; Freidson 1970, 2001; Johnson 1972; Burrage 1990; Torstendahl and Burrage 1990; Witz 1992; Evetts 2003, 2008; George 2013; Adams 2015). The study of professions has a long history, too complex to go into here; what is worth keeping in mind are the different meanings embodied in the word profession in the Anglo-American context and in the Continental European context. These two realms have been characterized by certain trends: on the Continent, the professionalization processes have been historically imposed from above, whereas in the Anglo-American context, the same professional groups activate processes from within (Mcclelland 1990). While the European model emphasizes the role of the administrative elites who gain positions through the fulfillment of

DOI: 10.4324/9781003165934-4

academic requirements, the Anglo-American model emphasizes the freedom of self-employed practitioners who independently control their working conditions (Collins 1990). However, in the last three decades, there have been some convergences between Anglo-American and European societies, favored by the spread of the American neoliberal model on the Continent (Svensson and Evetts 2010; Abbott 2018).

After a century of state-ruled capitalism, in Europe we have begun to witness a process in which the market progressively replaces state regulations (Albert 1991). In Italy, this process has involved many types of actions: flexibility of the labor market; outsourcing of services; cuts to public funding in many sectors, especially education, health, and welfare; reduction of state and territorial bodies; transformations in the management of services from public to private; managerialization in all public sectors; and the introduction of standardization and performance control systems. The legislative provisions concerning unregulated professions and the emergence of professions, such as the doula profession, are also included in this frame.

Given the social context, the constant evolution, and the limited usefulness of adopting a rigid definition of the concept of professions, I will focus on the processes that doulas are implementing, following the indication of Abbott: "[...] one could start by discussing exactly what a profession is. But the numbers of possible definitions are overwhelming ... To start with a definition is thus not to start at all" (1991:18).

Studying the doula profession

To study how the doula profession is developing, I chose to adopt a principal theoretical reference (Abbott 1988), integrating it with reflections from other authors (Elias 2007; Adams 2007) to build a framework capable of capturing the complexity of this ongoing process. Elias (2007) regards professions as specialized social functions put in place by some people in response to the needs of others; however, the emergence of a new occupation is not solely due to the emergence of new needs or new techniques, but to their interaction. It is a process of attempts and failures, in which professionals seek to match techniques or occupational institutions to people's needs. Conflicts and tensions involving professionals and professional groups, or factions engaged in providing solutions to emerging needs, determine the long-term development of the profession. Therefore, a profession, according to Elias, arises on the basis of an unsatisfied need, but also from the inability of preexisting institutions to provide solutions to emerging problems.

In the case of Italian doulas, the lack of social public policies for supporting mothers and families, the excessive medicalization of childbirth, and the lack of empathy from health professionals are the generating elements of the emergence of the profile. Doulas, who are engaged in attempts to meet the needs expressed by mothers and to remedy the shortcomings of the public welfare system, have activated training courses, founded associations, and undertaken paths to regulate this emergent profession, as described in Chapter 2. As Lisa, a doula, put it:

> The situation of the Italian women of today ... there is too much need of the doula ... because women are lonely, they no longer have families behind them because mothers work until old age, many times families move so they do not live in the city of origin, many times new mothers have to go back to work early so they need extra support again...

In Italy, as Lisa notes, there is a lack of a real social policy for the family (Saraceno 2003). Until a few decades ago, this situation was overcome thanks to family solidarity and the accompanying willingness to provide care and support. But in recent years, changes in social and economic dynamics have impeded the family network from supporting the pregnant or newborn mother, and consequently, new mothers need to look for support elsewhere. In the narratives of doulas, this dimension is described as a "void." Despite social and economic changes, public policies have not foreseen support paths for new mothers. For this reason, as doula Alba explains, doulas have developed and spread with the aim of filling this void:

> ... there is a distance, women complain about a great distance with the professionals who should take care of them, with doctors, gynecologists, midwives, complain about a lack of support, a lack of closeness, empathy, understanding, lament a loneliness that is something more than the loneliness given by the transformation of society.

This lack of empathy and closeness with health professionals is heavily present in the Italian realm. Pizzini (1999) notes that, through obstetric procedures, the "biomedical definition" is inscribed upon the physiological process of childbirth; that definition includes the hospital, the healthcare professionals, and the laboring woman. I see that biomedical definition of birth (Emerson 2008) as a defense strategy of maternity care professionals to block any emotion and anxiety they may feel in relation to birth as a complex biosocial and biomedical event. The midwife, whose tasks also include the emotional support of women, is in a position of subordination with respect to the physician that began with the hospitalization of birth (Spina 2014).

The biomedicalization of birth with its lack of empathy and compassion generates in the laboring woman the need for emotional support that used to be filled by other women who accompanied women in childbirth; thus, she looks for the satisfaction of her need to her network of family and friends—and now, to the doula. As Nina succinctly put it, "the doula perhaps exists because there is a void that they have created...because the history of medicalization has led to this."

For a century now, and especially over the last four decades, the progressive development of biomedicine has determined a process of hospitalization and medicalization from procreation to childbirth (Minicuci 1985; Pizzini 1985; Colombo et al. 1985; Bestetti et al. 2005; Davis-Floyd 2003, 2022). The daily life of human reproduction is in the hands of women, but its practice and control are in the hands of biomedicine—the privileged field of a professional elite (Pizzini 1999)—that produces and reproduces medicalization using technological equipment, since any biomedical act is considered to be more "scientific" when it is performed by or via a technological artifact (Regalia 1985). Since the moment pregnancy became instrumentally verifiable, the womb has become an area of intervention and control and the pregnant woman a uterine system for fetal supply (Duden 1991). The medicalization of the female body has been interpreted as the response of modernity to the need for social control and technological surveillance over women's reproductive activities (Jordan 1983; Davis Floyd 1997, 2003, 2022). The specialization of techniques, although it did aid in the reduction of maternal and perinatal mortality, appears to have contributed to the creation of a void, a detachment, not only related to the interaction between maternity care professionals and women, but also linked to technocratic practice itself. The delegation of childbirth and reproduction to the modern technologies employed by biomedicine, perhaps better referred to as "techno-medicine" (Davis-Floyd 2003, 2022), in order to monitor the state of health of the woman and the fetus, has led visual perception to dominate the other senses, so as to paralyze touch and smell, hearing (Duden 1991). This lack of contact, emphasized by detached and technologically mediated interactions, has generated the need for women to be seen, heard, and touched in precisely the ways that doulas do.

Desiring a formal recognition or, as defined by Abbott (1988), a *jurisdiction*, a profession demands that its cognitive and social structure be recognized through exclusive rights. Abbot considers that every profession is immersed in a system where different jurisdictions meet, clash, and, on some occasions, overlap. For this reason, he rejects the idea that the process of professionalization assumes a one-way path and invites the analysis of the contents of professional work and the efforts made by professionals belonging to the same professional group to affirm its jurisdiction.

An emerging profession may attempt to occupy an empty space or may overlap, at least partially, with an already occupied space. The doula occupies the empty space created by the lack of emotional and practical support during pregnancy, labor, and postpartum and her role and practice may sometimes overlap with that of other nearby professions. Only by considering the tensions and conflicts within the professional group and with neighboring occupational groups, it is possible to analyze and understand the processes that determine the new profession's development.

According to Abbott, jurisdiction is composed of two aspects: cultural and structural. Abbott states that a profession must first define its area of competence by building it culturally; for example, "fatness" must be transformed into the pathology of obesity and in this way, work is created for a professional who deals with this now-pathological problem. Any occupation that competes for a job through this type of cultural activity can be defined as a profession. For this reason, doula practice can be considered a profession, since it is culturally developing its area of competence (see Chapter 4), also defining its structural aspects through jurisdictional claims in the three arenas identified by Abbott (1988): the legal system, public opinion, and the workplace.

The public opinion arena refers to all communicative actions (articles published in newspapers, magazines, websites, and blogs) that have the function of sharing with the public some aspects and activities of the profession, attracting interest and disseminating professional values. In this arena, the professional group of doulas in Italy is very active, with several web pages, articles in national newspapers and magazines, blogs, etc. Despite differences in the trainings and in the approaches of the different doula associations (see Chapter 4), the professional group is very compact. When you read an interview with a doula, it always refers to the doula group as a whole; it is almost never specified whether the doula is part of an association or not, or if the doula has specific skills and specializations. Yet doing so would be extremely important to promoting a coherent professional profile, since the doula is not yet known by the majority of the Italian population.

The request for jurisdiction in the arena of the legal system, adapted to the Italian context as an arena of the state system, is expressed through the actions taken by emerging professionals to achieve state regulation. In the case of doulas, this refers to the attempt to obtain a statal recognition of their activities, as required by Law no. 4 of 2013. However, the request for jurisdiction in this arena appears to be closely linked to the jurisdiction relating to the workplace, since it is in the field that the control of tasks is defined. Who controls and supervises the work and who defines the roles? In the case of doulas, these tasks have thus far been carried out by the main doulas' associations.

I find it important to emphasize the social and cultural control embodied by the professional jurisdiction. Social and cultural control is in fact exclusive: a profession can choose to found associations, create schools, newsletters, and magazines, but it cannot occupy a jurisdiction without finding a vacant space or without fighting to create one, as chiropractors had to do in the U.S.A.: it took them around 50 years to generate that space and create their jurisdiction over it. Since the jurisdiction is—or seeks to be—exclusive, the professions constitute an interdependent system: the movement of one inevitably involves others. The contention over the same or overlapping jurisdictions by two or more occupations[1] generates interprofessional conflict—an endemic characteristic in the system of professions.

---

1 Such as medical doctors (MDs) and doctors of osteopathy (DOs) in the U.S.A.

In Chapter 6, I will analyze the tensions between the professional groups of doulas and the professional groups of midwives to explore how they are defining their jurisdictions. However, in certain circumstances, professional development can take place through interprofessional cooperation and collaboration (Adams 2007). The conditions for effective collaboration identified by Adams include a similarity in the size, mentality/perspective, and legal status of the professional groups involved. These conditions are particularly interesting for my purposes here, as they expand my toolkit for investigating relationships between doulas and midwives (see Chapter 6).

Doulas are care professionals

The study of the doula profile has stimulated the adoption of different interpretive lenses; among these, the "care approach" seems to best capture the specific characteristics of the figure: "This is the work of care: interpreting and defining needs; if one succeeds, satisfying desires" (Balbo 2008: 61; my translation). Balbo's words express the essence of doulas' work. Thus, I have approached the topic using the "ethics of care" as the most comprehensive theoretical elaboration for the interpretation of the doula profile.

The numerous debates surrounding the ethics of care have been prompted largely by the work of psychologist Carol Gilligan (1982) on the differences she noted in the development of the moral judgment of girls and boys and, subsequently, has concerned different disciplines—sociology, anthropology, economics, political theory, philosophy—committed to shedding light on the complexities of the dimensions of this approach.

The elements that characterize the ethics of care, according to Sevenhuijsen (2000, 2003), are the intersubjective responsibilities between who gives and who receives care, and their relational qualities. Reflections on the ethics of care also allow us to definitively overcome the traditional interpretation that framed the social care professions as extensions of maternal and/or feminine skills. This does not mean that caregiving professionals should detach themselves from their own experiences, but instead that they should integrate those embodied resources and skills with their professional knowledge (Bimbi 1995, 2000). In other words, the ethics of care underlines the need to deconstruct the walls of "those in need" with respect to "those who hold the techniques to help them"—to create a system of relations that binds those who lend help to those who need help. Kittay (1999, 2001) makes explicit reference to the figure of the doula to develop the principle of *doulia*. Expanding the notion of doula, with the term *doulia*, Kittay indexes the public responsibility to provide support for the caregiver so that the caregiver can give care without depleting herself and her resources. Just as the doula takes care of the mother, and the mother takes care of her child, following the principle of *doulia* and the ethics of care approach, someone must take care of the doula. This principle of reciprocity can be identified for the whole society as an association that lasts from generation to generation.

The model of doula care has therefore been used as a paradigm for developing a system of care that would weave a network of reciprocity for the entire society, since it embodies a dimension of innovative and mutual care:

> The doula is a caregiver: she takes care of the emotional, relational needs of a woman during a very important time ... from a relational point of view but sometimes also from a material point of view—I cook a pasta for you, I vacuum ...
>
> (Mara)

> ... be there without overwhelming, be there ... I'm the doula, I'm a doula... I mean, I don't have to play the role, I *am* the role. For me perhaps the most important thing is to be a demonstration always, so a profession that is not something that you wear but that you are—you become what you represent.
>
> (Alda)

Attention to needs, the will to take care of other individuals, the incorporation of an attitude that does not refer to a set of techniques but rather to a rational moral disposition (Sevenhuijsen 2000) are characteristics of the doula profile, as interlocutors show. As Sciurba (2015) points out, quoting Gilligan (1982), the ethics of care with their attention to voice—to the fact that everyone has a voice and that voice must be heard and understood—and to relationships, constitute the proper ethics of a democratic society.

A further significant contribution comes from the work of Tronto (1993). This author considers care as a continuous process, and divides it into four phases:

- caring about, which presupposes the moral quality of attention to others and the recognition that care is necessary;
- taking care of, which involves taking responsibility for the needs of others and identifying strategies and actions to meet those needs;
- care giving, which involves the concrete satisfaction of needs, through the actions identified at the time of taking responsibility;
- care receiving, which entails the feedback of the one who has received care.

Care is therefore a process and a practice; it involves both action and reflection. According to interlocutors, this is how doulas operate.

To avoid the risk of care professions emptying themselves of the emotional dimension, it is necessary to develop a professional model that places the caregiver at the center of the care work: the caregiver gives care but needs to receive care as well. The embodiment of a professional attitude that requires considerable emotional involvement is one of the biggest challenges for care professionals, which among other professions is generally solved via operationalizing an emotional detachment (Colombo 2004; Maluccelli 2007). Yet considering the emotional specificities of doula work, I can affirm that this kind of detachment cannot be included in its practice. It is for this reason that doulas carefully pay attention to their own emotionality. From the narratives of interlocutors, it emerges that attention to themselves has become a fundamental strategy for their professional identity: to take care of themselves in order to take care of others. Rita described how doulas take care of each other:

> Meeting and discussing is important for us ... we do it every 15 days, sometimes we talk about our own business, how are the children ... other times when there are cases to be discussed we discussed them ...

The ways in which doulas manifest their needs and receive support from their peers are varied: through meetings with colleagues, as showed in the Figure 3.1 and as Rita described; through virtual interactions with members of the same association; through meetings with trainers who continue to offer availability even when the training is finished; or through moments of leisure and relaxation. For example, one interlocutor included in her marketing materials a "Frequently Asked Questions" section, in which she explains that her fee includes shiatsu treatments for herself, since to make

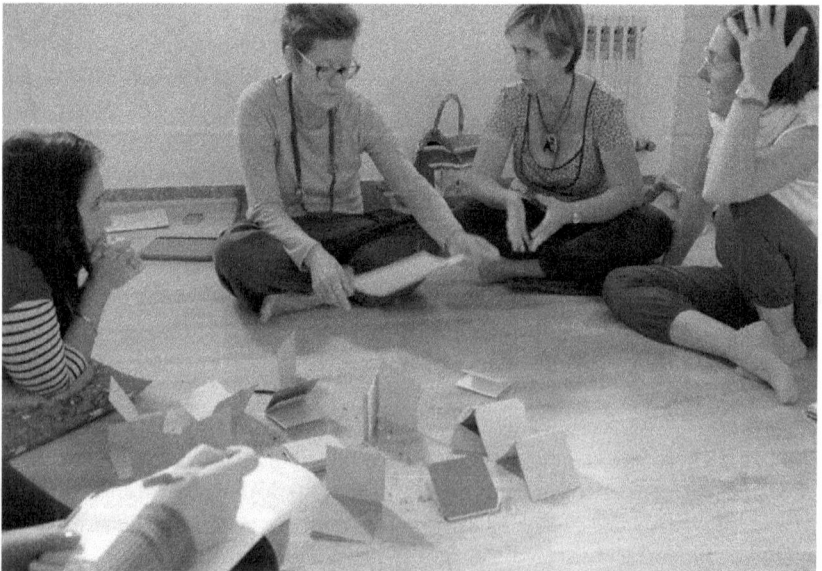

Figure 3.1 Doulas of the Association Le Lune Allegre supporting each other and creating activities for mothers.

Source: Photograph by Licia Valso.

the mother feel good, the doula has to feel good too. Although the strategies and tools adopted by doulas to take care of themselves differ, it is essential in their professional practice to foresee moments of sharing, of relaxation, and of support in order to counter the wear and tear that their high level of emotional involvement can cause.

Doulas and medical excess: over-intervention in birth

The study of the doula profession and the contexts in which it operates has required the widening of my gaze to the biomedical field and to the excess (Abbott 2014) of biomedicalization that has characterized the perinatal period over the last decades (Ehrenreich and English 1977; Johanson et al. 2002; Anderson 2004). Medicalization in this area has included, among many other interventions, induction of labor, epidural use, and excessive use of cesarean sections; these interventions enact the technocratic paradigm of birth (Davis-Floyd 2001, 2018). But there is also an opposing movement that promotes natural childbirth (Lowenberg and Davis 1994; Page 2001; Mansfiel 2008) and coincides with the humanistic and holistic paradigms as delineated by Davis Floyd (2001, 2018, 2022) and as described below.

The technocratic paradigm began to develop with the transfer to hospital of childbirth in tandem with the transition from the female world of midwives to the male world of obstetricians (Sbisà 1992; Lombardi and Pizzini 2004) who for decades now have attributed great importance to the use of modern visual technologies [ultrasounds, cardiotopography (electronic fetal monitoring), X-rays, etc.] to diagnose the state of health of the woman and the fetus. The female body thus becomes the nature over which male culture exercises its dominion (Pitch 2006), both practical and symbolic (Romito and Chatelanat 1985; Bourdieu 1998). These elements constitute the indicators that sanction the passage of childbirth from a biosocial to a biomedical event. Conrad (1992: 209) defined medicalization as that process by which "non-medical problems are defined and treated as medical problems, often in terms of disease and disorder," and in this sense, pregnancy and childbirth are emblematic cases. They are physiological processes that are defined as pathological risks under the influence of technocratic biomedical ideology (Oakley and Houd 1990; Davis-Floyd 2022).

Multiple scholars (see, e.g., Oakley 1992; Martin 2001; Johanson et al. 2002) have criticized the control of the birth process and of women in labor by biomedical maternity care professionals. Moreover, research has revealed that the use of technology weakens women's control of the birth process (Davis Floyd 1994, 2003; Martin 2001). It is precisely the excess of confidence (Abbott 2014) in clinical examinations and diagnoses, instead of in clinical observation and a trust relationship between doctors and pregnant women, that enables obstetricians to define childbearing as a potentially pathological process. Nevertheless, some researchers (Sargent and Stark 1989; Lazarus 1994; Davis-Floyd 2003, 2022) have pointed out that many women actively seek medical supervision for the unpredictable event of childbirth.

In recent decades, biomedicine has witnessed the emergence of unconventional therapeutic practices (homeopathy, osteopathy, chiropractic, etc.), and the development of diagnostic and treatment models born in non-Western cultures, such as acupuncture, Ayurvedic medicine, shiatsu, etc. (Colombo 2003). The advent of these "alternative" or "complementary" models of medicine, combined with the transformations in the organization of the healthcare system, the spread of both biomedical and "alternative" knowledge through the mass media, and the increase in informed patients has marked a partial decline in the authority of the biomedical profession and the introduction of the concept of the "de-medicalization of birth." In this sense, in the literature on childbirth, numerous studies have highlighted the active roles of mothers and fathers in biomedical–patient interaction and in the decision-making processes regarding pregnancy and childbirth (Shorten et al. 2005; van der Hulst et al. 2007).

To understand the debates on medicalization, de-medicalization needs to be contextualized (Ballard and Elston, 2005). In other words, de-medicalization is always de-medicalization from over-medicalization. This concept often emerged in my interviews with doulas, and to deepen this dimension, in the next section, I will analyze the models of assistance to pregnancy and childbirth using the paradigms proposed by Davis-Floyd (2001, 2018)—the technocratic, humanistic, and holistic models of birth.

Which paradigm(s) do doulas use to support mothers?

Robbie Davis Floyd has identified three paradigms of childbirth assistance that characterize Western societies: technocratic, humanistic, and holistic (2001, 2018). According to Davis-Floyd, the technocratic paradigm is the ideology that underlies the Western techno-medical system and reflects the values of technocratic societies. Davis-Floyd (2018:4) defines a "technocracy" as "a hierarchical, bureaucratic, capitalistic, and (still) patriarchal society organized around an ideology of the importance of the development of ever-higher technologies and the global flow of information through such technologies." She notes that the technocratic model of birth reflects and enacts the core values of technocratic societies, just as all birthways reflect and enact the core values of their respective cultures. According to her, the technocratic model is based on the conceptual separation of mind and body, treats the body as if it were a machine, and is supposedly anchored in science, implemented with a high use of technology, and developed through patriarchal institutions in a profit-oriented context. In this model, technology reigns supreme and, accordingly, the need to technologically intervene from the outside has justified for decades many medical procedures executed routinely, not for scientific, but for cultural reasons having to do with what Davis-Floyd calls the technocratic "supervaluation" of high technology. This scholar (Davis-Floyd 2022) has also interpreted standard obstetric procedures as nonevidence-based rituals that enact and transmit technocratic core values and that provide a sense of cultural safety to many childbearers, as rituals are so good at doing (Pizzini 1999).

The humanistic paradigm emerged as an effort to mitigate the excesses of the cold and impersonal technocratic treatment of birth and was initially developed by nurses, some obstetricians, and other health professionals with the aim of reforming the system from within. The supporters of this approach aim to humanize techno-medicine so that it becomes relational, compassionate, oriented to collaboration between practitioner and patient, and able to redistribute the responsibilities, giving more agency to the woman as the protagonist of her own birth. In this model, the body is viewed and treated as an affective organism, not as a machine, and mind and body are viewed as connected—meaning that what happens in the mind and the emotions can affect labor progress. *Listening to women* and developing caring relationships with them are two of humanism's primary values. The humanistic model as Davis-Floyd defines it does encompass the judicious use of interventive technologies when truly needed, in what Cheyney and Davis-Floyd (2020a, 2020b, 2021) call RARTRW care—"the right amount at the right time in the right way." These authors propose RARTRW care as the humanistic solution to the TMTS ("too much too soon") or TLTL ("too little too late") dichotomy that characterizes the application of the technocratic model in many countries—low- and high-resource alike (Miller et al. 2016). The well-off in any country tend to receive TMTS care—too many interventions implemented too soon in the birthing process, while TLTL—too few needed interventions given too late in the processes of labor and birth—generally characterizes the care received by the poor and marginalized (ibid.) The presence of the doula can help to ensure the provision of humanistic, RARTRW care.

The holistic paradigm also encompasses RARTRW care, yet makes a conceptual leap far beyond that to consider mind, body, and spirit as constituting a unified energy field in constant interaction with other energy fields. Thus, under this model, paying attention to the energy in the room is essential: "change the energy, change the outcome." This holistic model, which generally characterizes what Cheyney (2011) calls "the system-challenging praxis" of births at home and in freestanding birth centers, also encompasses various types of complementary approaches (Colombo and Rebughini 2003), many of which are energy-based, such as homeopathy, Reiki, acupuncture, and many others. Those who do not grasp the existence of that intangible phenomenon called "energy" consider such healing systems to be "quackery." One of the reasons many childbearers and others reject the holistic approach is that it requires taking personal responsibility for one's health and well-being by making long-term changes in lifestyle, and for one's birth—a responsibility that, as Davis-Floyd (2003, 2018, 2022) has shown, many prefer to delegate to their biomedical doctors. That is one of the reasons why it is the humanistic paradigm that has made the greatest inroads into the techno-medical management of birth: *all* childbearers wish to be treated with the kindness, respect, and compassion that the humanistic approach entails. Doulas have key roles to play in the humanization of birth.

From the analysis of interviews with the doulas emerged diversified positionings that encompass elements of both the humanistic and the holistic paradigms. The technocratic paradigm, also termed "the medical model" (Rothman 2001; van Teijlingen 2005), which falls within the broader conceptual framework of techno-medicalization (Parson 1950; Zola 1972; Illich 1976; Conrad 1992; Maturo and Conrad 2009; Christiaens and van Teijlingen 2009), emerges as the approach to be countered:

> You have to understand when medicine is at the service of well-being and when instead it is ritualized within institutions, so it becomes a repetition of patterns of power and not true service to women or people in general ... The problem is that the medical world tries to treat pregnancy and childbirth as it treats other areas of medicine, and this cannot be ... the obstetrics ward is not the same as the orthopedics one, but they are in the same hospital, and they tend to work in the same way, with standards, with protocols, with doctors who do not see the person but see the pathology.
>
> (Mara)

> I believe that much of the medicalization of childbirth comes from the will to silence us, to take away the ability to believe in what we know how to do and that we have always done ... an impoverishment of the capacity of the woman, to make, to be, to create—and this impoverishes the woman not only in the moment of the delivery but in all her existence.
>
> (Emma)

> Medicalization is like it puts you in trouble when you're not there, doctors see you in categories ... medicalization takes away more than what it gives, then of course it saves people, but it would be better a little slowing down ... You go to the hospital and you fit into a protocol, that is, everything that is your perception, your motherhood history, your mother's opinion is not contemplated, the subjectivity of the person is not contemplated... I think it's an important thing in a healing process.
>
> (Leda)

Nevertheless, doulas maintain a neutral approach toward medicalization during their practices with mothers, as Alba stated:

> ... I'm not a non-medicalized birth activist when I'm doula; if a mother tells me she's afraid of giving birth and wants to do a scheduled C-section, I'll ask her what drives her to do this, but I don't do non-medicalization propaganda.

In contrast, Iris considered medicalization as a tool. Mothers-to-be should receive accurate information about all processes and hospital protocols, in order to make conscious decisions about what is better for themselves. Iris stated, "I think that medicalization must be an instrument in the hands of the mother. Of course, if she chooses a C-section after being informed and makes an aware choice, well, I welcome that... mothers must have tools."

The standardization/ritualization of obstetric procedures, the use of diagnostic and interventive technologies, and the objectification and pathologization of the experiences of pregnancy and childbirth emerge in doulas' narratives as the aspects that must be countered, because they conceal their true (and hidden) objective of annihilating the subjectivity of the woman through the control of her body. The medicalization of the female body has been interpreted as the response of modernity to the technocratic need for social control over women's reproductive activities (Jordan 1983; Davis-Floyd and Sargent 1997).

Research from various academic disciplines has criticized the expansion of the technocratic model in childbirth, suggesting that the use of technology leads to alienation through the weakening of control of the birth process by women (Martin 2001); technological procedures, especially when unwanted, often have a negative impact on psychological well-being (Fisher et al. 1997) and on mother–child interaction (Rowe-Murray and Fisher 2001); an invasive birth experience, especially in the case of cesarean, generates a greater possibility of psychological suffering in women (Ryding et al. 1997; Wijma et al. 2002). The humanistic and holistic models, on the other hand, give greater decision-making autonomy to the mother, often resulting in satisfaction with her childbirth experience (Hundley et al. 1997; Christiaens and Bracke 2007) and in stimulating self-confidence and self-care (Thachuk 2007): an empowered birthgiver becomes an empowered mother.

However, a controversial aspect emerges from my interviews with doulas: the need of most women to rely on techno-medicine to ensure that the processes of pregnancy and childbirth end with a positive outcome— meaning a physically healthy baby and mother. This aspect has also been noted by some authors who, through their research, have confirmed the satisfaction of some women in adhering to the technocratic model, as, again, it gives them a sense of safety (Lazarus 1994; Fox and Worts 1999; Davis-Floyd 2003, 2022). In order to understand this contradiction, Fox and Worts (1999) proposed looking at the social contexts and circumstances in which women give birth. Their research findings show that women want and adhere to the technocratic model the most when the social support that surrounds them is minimal. In this way, they seek to ensure the well-being of the newborn and to make themselves into patients, as in that role, they receive needed attention from healthcare professionals that they cannot get anywhere else. In contrast, women who can rely on a solid family and friendship network and/or a trusted doula have shown less propensity to embrace the technocratic model. Fox and Worts (ibid.) conclude that in order to take control of pregnancy and childbirth and to get their practitioners to adhere to a humanistic model of care, women need substantial social support.

Doulas aim to support the woman and the family and offer the social support that Fox and Worts recognize as essential. Childbearers who adhere to the technocratic model generally do not seek doula care, as their need for support is already satisfied by technocratic practitioners. If a woman who adheres to the technocratic model does want a doula, then that doula will not deny her support and will seek through dialogue to stimulate reflection. Moreover, doulas aim to promote a kind of body reappropriation by women. The connection and integration of the body, mind, and spirit are opposed to the segmentation of body parts generated by the technocratic model. Following interlocutors' narratives, I can see that women who adhere to the technocratic model have incorporated that habitus, and it is only through empowerment processes that such women can regain the power of self-determination, which, according to Emma:

> ... is what I call my personal neo-feminism ... for me feminism is not we pretend to be men and we become like them. Absolutely, for me feminism starts from repossessing our childbirth, repossessing our choices, our strength ... give value to our being women, full of power and choice.

Conclusion

The aim of this chapter has been to compare and contrast theoretical approaches coming from different points of observation to analyze the doula profession. Starting from a comparison between the Continental European and the Anglo-American traditions regarding the professions, I moved on to the insights and reflections of various scholars and to perspectives from the sociology of professions, from the feminists and philosophical literature, and from the health and reproduction sectors of sociology and anthropology. The insights I obtained from this literature enable me to affirm that the doula is a social care profession. But this profession does not yet have a name. Midwives engage in a profession called "midwifery"; obstetricians in a profession called "obstetrics"; nurses in a profession called "nursing." There is no such name for what I thus must call "the doula profession." Yet perhaps the time is ripe to take a step forward and introduce the word *doulaing* (as in "nurs*ing*") to name the doula profession. In the Italian context, doulas are used to a jargon full of neologisms to name their work. *Doulare* is the infinitive form of the verb that describes the activity of doulas. *Doulaggio* is the noun to describe the service. *Doulesco* is the adjective used to describe everything that can reflect the typical doula approach and style (see Chapter 4). These words are not yet included in the Italian dictionary, but they probably will be in the future. The word "doula" appeared in the Italian dictionary for the first time in 2015.

Through their professional activities, doulas aim to fill emotional and institutional voids by empowering women and resituating them as the protagonists of their births. Doula practice is based on an innovative model of care that is ultimately capable of weaving a network of reciprocity for the entire society. Embodying and promoting this care style, doulas wish to transform the cultural, technocratic approach to maternity care into a humanistic approach that encompasses relationship-based care and keeps the woman at the center of that care.

In Chapter 4, I will address the characteristics of the doula profession, the paths to becoming a doula in Italy, and the specificities of doula practices.

4 Doula training

As described in Chapter 3, the professions aim to provide solutions to human problems through the implementation of expert services. The level of specialization of these services may vary in relation to the type of problem, society, or historical context (Abbott 1988). The cultural basis of a profession is a system of knowledge that formalizes the skills that characterize it. The abstract corpus that underpins the professional knowledge system is generally organized through classifications, rationally structured, and logically consistent. In most professions, classification work is carried out by the professional association that has the task of demonstrating the rigor and scientific nature of the work of the profession in question. To study the doula profile, it is necessary to investigate the system of knowledge in which doula work is anchored. To analyze that knowledge system, I begin by examining the elements characterizing the training paths to become doulas in Italy, after first investigating some of the reasons why some women choose to become doulas.

The choice to become a doula

In the Italian context, the figure of the doula is unknown to most of the population; awareness of doulas' existence and work seems confined to the niche of professionals working in maternity care and to some women who have experienced giving birth in recent years. In the narrations of the interlocutors, the profile's discovery is described as a casual episode, fortuitous and a generator of surprise; as Nina put it:

Out of nowhere came this figure, doula, so puff!

The interlocutors encountered the doula through the media (Internet, books, or magazines), friends, family, or through maternity care professionals encountered during pregnancy or immediately after. Often, once the profile is known, the interlocutors say that they have carried out online research to deepen their understanding of doula work and to decide whether or not to undertake doula training:

DOI: 10.4324/9781003165934-5

I found myself in a situation where so many mothers find themselves, without help ... I had to deal with it all by myself, and from this very, very strong experience of early motherhood came the idea of doing something for women in my condition.

(Nina)

... I experienced in my own skin the loneliness and despair of my mother, a bit this idea of "mothering the mother." I think was born when I was very small ... then anyway I got pregnant ... and even there the loneliness I felt was not physical ... but psychological loneliness, yes.

(Zita)

From these interlocutors' narrations, it emerged that their interest in becoming a doula arises more from personal motivations than from the need or desire to undertake a professional activity. A passion for the topics related to *maternage* or an unsatisfactory personal birthing experience, sometimes traumatic, represents the most common situations that have encouraged women to become doulas.

Training paths

In Italy, as described in Chapter 2, doulas are governed by law number 4 of 2013, "Provisions on unregulated professions"; therefore, doula practices and training paths are not regulated by state norms but are fully open to market rules and structuring by private organizations. The original doula trainings in Italy were created by their inventors—Emanuela Geraci and Maria Grazia Biagini for Mondo Doula, and Laura Verdi for Adi—merging competence and skills they acquired through trainings in counseling, midwifery, and education with desires, reflections, wishes, and personal insights. Generally, in the Italian context, when I talk about doulas, I mean full spectrum doulas, trained to support women during pregnancy, labor, and the postpartum period.

In 2014, when this research project was developed, the Italian associations that offered doula training courses were Mondo Doula, Mammadoula, Adi-Associazione Doule Italia, Progetto Primo Respiro, and 13doule, whereas by May 2021, only Mondo Doula, Mammadoula, Adi, and Progetto Primo Respiro promoted doula trainings on their websites. A new training called "Accademia delle doule" started at this time of writing—September 2021.

Doulas' associations that offer trainings have equipped themselves with a professional structure: nine or more weekends of training, developed over nine or more months, during which, through the adoption and development of a relational approach, the main themes concerning motherhood are addressed. Ample space is reserved for introspective work, to analyze personal experiences as mothers or daughters, in order to avoid projecting their personal issues onto their clients. The duration of the training mirrors the duration of pregnancy, since to come into the world as a doula means to be "reborn" as a woman. Becoming a doula is a transformative process that requires time, patience, and reflexivity.

To be able to access doula training, the requirement is the same for all the schools: motivation. Access is open to anyone who demonstrates, after an interview with one of the trainers and/or organizers of the courses, to have understood the characteristics of the doula profile and to be willing to undertake an introspective path to draw on personal resources and experiences to manage and care relationships. Four associations have an additional requirement: being a woman. The only association that guarantees access to men is Mondo Doula, which considers that a motivated and willing man can be an excellent resource for supporting mothers, fathers, and families. Doula trainings attract women from extremely heterogeneous social, cultural, and educational backgrounds. The cost of the training is defined by each school and is between €900 and €1750 for the entire first-year course. The School of Laura Verdi, created by Adi-Association Doule Italia, presents a substantial difference from the other schools: it provides a first year of training to become a postpartum doula and a second year of training to become a labor and birth doula.

During the training courses, students are asked to undertake one or more internships with volunteer women during pregnancy, labor, or postpartum; Progetto Primo Respiro provides the opportunity to carry out the internship at the training institution, while Accademia delle doule offers internships in healthcare facilities, including abroad. During the internship, doula students have to identify a mother, who can be a friend, a relative, or anyone available, and support her as if they were professional doulas. The mother is aware that the doula is still a student and accepts that because the support is free-of-charge, while the doula can test herself in the field, implementing what she learned during the training. Throughout the internship, the doula is supervised by trainers and tutors, who support her along the entire path.

At the end of the internship, students have to write a report. Each school provides a bibliography of books to be studied; asks the students to write reports about some of those books or about other topics that interest them; oversees a final exam; and requires paid supervision (depending on the schools) with the course trainers. By "supervision," I mean one or more meetings (depending on the specific situation and need) with one trainer, who is a psychologist, counselor, or doula expert, to overcome any difficulties encountered once the doula is in professional practice.

Each school designs the final exam in a different way: through writing a paper or taking a written exam, and/or role playing. The role playing usually involves two students. The trainer invites one student to play the mother's role with a specific problem, while the aspiring doula has to show how she would support this mother, overcoming the difficulty. Or, for example, Mammadoula requires the student to draft a critical review of the mandatory texts and to map the structures and services related to motherhood available in the city of the trainee. At the end of the training, the assessment of students is carried out by the teaching staff of the school. A diploma is delivered to all participants, excepting those candidates considered not suitable to serve as a doula. In the case of Mammadoula, the teaching staff can decide not to give her a diploma; in the case of Mondo Doula, the trainers can suggest implementing an introspective/psychological path to become able to manage a care relationship.

When the basic training has been completed, most respondents say they have identified areas of specific interest and have attended—or plan to attend—other trainings to expand their knowledge. Each association offers ongoing seminars and workshops; Adi, Progetto Primo Respiro, Mammadoula, and Mondo Doula require their graduates to participate in these ongoing trainings, seminars, and workshops for continuing education. Although there are some differences among the associations, the teaching staff responsible for training is generally made up of doulas, counselors, psychologists, IBCLCs (International Board Certified Lactation Consultants), and midwives; often trainers are members of the association board.

To understand the system of knowledge and skills that characterize the doula profile, I will analyze the contents of the training programs of the associations Mondo Doula, Mammadoula, and Progetto Primo Respiro as found on the Internet. The programs of Adi and 13 doule were not published online and thus are not discussed herein. From my analysis of the objectives of the three training courses emerges a single, fundamental, convergence: the desire to deal with the theme of motherhood, bringing it back to the center of public debate, and through the training to become able to support women and families in a personalized and flexible way.

For Mondo Doula, the doula profession is a relational one and the school, rather than teaching a series of techniques, aims to develop the embodiment of a caring style and a willingness to make oneself available for others. To legitimize the profile, the training courses assemble knowledge and skills in original ways; some of these may be shared with other professions but are attributed new meaning in the context of doula work. Mondo Doula is defined as a professional association and considers the doula as a "social professional." The objectives proposed by Mammadoula are concisely described and do not refer to the professional character of the doula profile. However, even though Mammadoula does not use the word "professional," some aspects of its training program, which I will specify later on, demonstrate the professional attitudes of this association's approach and training. Progetto Primo Respiro defines the doula as a woman who has experience, preparation, and aptitude in supporting mothers and mothers-to-be. This school does not define the doula as a professional, even though it is explicit that doulas can work professionally according to law 4/2013. The differentiation in the objectives of each school illustrates the different visions held by these associations and the difficulties in finding a shared agreement among them in the process of defining the doula profession.

To analyze the trainings, I will organize their contents into disciplinary areas that I have identified to explicate the features of the doula profile. To do so, I have deconstructed the contents of each training as these appear on their respective websites. My analysis of the training programs of the three associations highlights two macro training arenas: the arena of practical skills and the arena of relational and emotional skills.

Practical skills

In the arena of practical skills, I have identified six primary topics: (1) historical, social, and professional doula profile and context; (2) physiological and social elements of the perinatal period; (3) techniques and practices; (4) communication elements; (5) social context and professional networking; (6) marketing and client management. The doula trainings appear to follow a circular process: one starts from the context, learns the ideology and the characterizing tools of the doula, and returns to the context to propose herself to the market.

Historical, social, and professional doula profile and contexts

In the initial part of the course, the schools deal with issues aimed at defining the problem that generated the birth of the doula, considering its historical, social, and professional contexts. There is similarity between the contents of the trainings given by Mondo Doula and Mammadoula: both associations frame the figure from an historical and social point of view, define the boundaries between the doula and other maternity care professions, and deepen students' understandings of the legal framework into which the doula is inserted. The Progetto Primo Respiro training appears to focus exclusively on the historical and social aspects of the doula, not considering the professional environment into which the doula fits nor the legal framework that governs it. The absence of these aspects confirms what is stated in the objectives of the course: the trainers of Progetto Primo Respiro do not consider the doula from a professional point of view but rather imagine her role as exclusively social: the doula as a supportive figure, an extension of the family and friend network, but not a birth professional.

Physiological and social elements of the perinatal period

The next dimension of the training courses concerns information related to the physiology of pregnancy, childbirth, and the postpartum period, and the contexts into which these phases of life are integrated. The programs of the three associations share some similarities, yet differ in other aspects. Mondo Doula and Progetto Primo Respiro provide training in the physiology of pregnancy and birth, while Mammadoula does not. This choice seems dictated by the desire for the doula not to deal with birth physiology, since the competent, related professional in that arena is the midwife. Not considering these aspects relevant to the training manifests Mammadoula's intention to draw a clear boundary between the competencies of doulas and those of midwives, and to avoid fueling the accusations of abuse of the midwifery profession.

Aspects that unite these programs concern the physiology of breastfeeding, bonding, the mother–baby relationship, and the nourishment of the newborn: it seems clear that a doula must be trained in how to support the feeding of the newborn, from breastfeeding to weaning. In Mondo Doula and Mammadoula, the breastfeeding training is based on the WHO–UNICEF course. In 2002, two United Nations agencies jointly drew up a global strategy—the Baby-friendly Hospital Initiative (BFHI)—for the feeding of infants and children, with the aim of bringing the world's attention to the effects of food practices, nutritional status, growth and development, health and, ultimately, the survival of infants and children. This strategy is based on the importance of nutrition in the first months and years of life, and on the decisive role that exclusive breastfeeding plays in the first six months (WHO 2006). Within the strategy, WHO and UNICEF have identified the need for adequate and up-to-date training of support figures for the new mother, and it is for this reason that the two schools decided to introduce this specific training in the 10 Steps of the BFHI.

All three training courses investigate some aspects that can complicate pregnancy and compromise its success: Mammadoula addresses the issues of spontaneous or voluntary abortion, mourning, prematurity, and disability; Mondo Doula treats the theme of perinatal mourning; Progetto Primo Respiro treats the themes of loss and trauma. The fact that these aspects are engaged in by all three schools emphasizes that the competence of the doula should include the ability to support a woman and her family even in complex and/or tragic moments.

Mondo Doula is the only association to include in its program the topic of the placenta and the symbolic value that it can have. The hospitalization of birth resulted in a loss of meaning compared to the value that the placenta and the umbilical cord had in the past. Ranisio (1998), who carried out a research project regarding the transformations that occurred in the beliefs, practices, and rituals of childbirth in the social and cultural context of southern Italy during the 1950s, points out that both the umbilical cord and the placenta were closely linked to the life of the child and mother. For example, in some areas close to Naples, the umbilical cord was attributed a life force that could facilitate baby growth. The umbilical cord was dried and then burned in the hearth at the beginning or at the end of the lunch during festivities, when the whole family was gathered at the table, to wish the newborn to be always present at such family banquets. This custom responded to the need to strengthen family ties with the newborn, sanctioning his/her entry into the group and propitiating his/her destiny. About the placenta, the connection between the maternal body and the placenta could be reaffirmed on the symbolic plane with the attribution to it of particular powers and breastmilk-enhancing properties, which ethnomedical studies later confirmed (Scarpa 1988, Lim 2014). The fact that childbearers usually no longer see their placentas, nor know where they end up, does not allow women and their families to attribute any vitality or meaning to this life-giving organ through which they could exercise symbolic control. The attention to the placenta and practices such as "lotus birth"— which consists of not cutting the umbilical cord, allowing the newborn to remain attached to his/her placenta until, after 2–10 days, the cord naturally separates from the newborn's navel—manifests a will to reappropriate the rituals of embodiment that the hospitalization of the birth has done away with (Cheyney 2011). Lotus birth can be done in homebirth and in a few hospitals; others don't allow it. Some hospitals do allow a "mini-lotus" birth, which consists of keeping the placenta attached for two hours, with the mother and baby skin-to-skin.

Techniques and practices: the birth plan

In the field of techniques and practices, I found a similarity in the training programs of Mammadoula and Mondo Doula about practices regarding the support of pregnant women and during labor. During pregnancy, tools such as the "birth plan" (not explained in the online program of Mammadoula but mentioned during the interviews) or the organization of a "Blessingway" are occasions for reflection on childbirth that the doula proposes to the client. The birth plan consists of a list of desires for her labor and birth that the woman writes and presents to the hospital/birth center where she decides to give birth. Through helping the pregnant woman to create her birth plan, the doula aims to stimulate a reflective process regarding the event that the client is about to live. The aspects addressed in the birth plan are connected to the different places where the client can give birth (hospital, freestanding birth center, home); the different hospitals present in her region; their operational protocols related to the use of analgesia; labor induction; the percentages of vaginal births and cesarean sections; the waiting time for cutting the umbilical cord; the possibility of collecting cord blood; the possibility of allowing the family to take the placenta home; the possibility of having a VBAC (vaginal birth after cesarean); and in general all those aspects that may physiologically affect the birth. Usually, the woman presents the birth plan indicating the procedures that she wishes and those she doesn't to the facility she has chosen. She discusses her birth plan with the midwife board or with the head of the department of obstetrics and gynecology and asks for its inclusion in her personal file. Hospital personnel often completely ignore these birth plans, yet, as Leda said, "the birth plan that we use is just a tool to feel strong … If you know you can present something like that, you feel that your body is in your hands too." From the accounts of doulas, it emerges that the birth plan constitutes an occasion to reflect on the coming labor and birth, but above all it offers the possibility of a reappropriation of childbirth by childbearers—a means of taking back control from the obstetric profession, which officially is the only discipline allowed to be in charge of childbirth (Pizzini 1999).

Techniques and practices: the Blessingway

The Blessingway—a ceremony originally created by the Navajo of the US Southwest as part of a longer puberty rite for girls that has been widely appropriated in the U.S.A. and elsewhere and transformed into a celebration of impending motherhood—is described by doulas as a party, a ceremony, a meeting where the pregnant woman gathers together with her closest relatives and friends. The aim of the Blessingway, organized a few weeks before the due date and usually carried out at her home or in another place dear to her, is to create a "sacred and safe environment where a mother-to-be can explore the challenges and joys that lie before her as she approaches birthing and mothering" (Cortlund et al. 2006:3). During the gathering, the participants take care of the future mother through massages, giving flowers and/or creating a flower crown to be placed on the pregnant woman's head, decorating her belly with henna or other types of colors, making a belly casting as in Figure 4.1 and 4.2, creating pearl necklaces or bracelets, sharing food, and in general being willing to accept any request that the

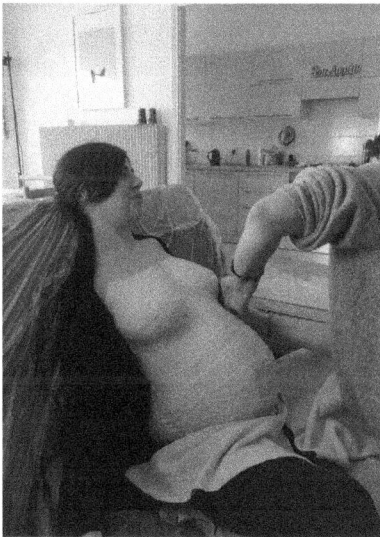

Figure 4.1 A doula doing a belly casting with a pregnant mom.
Source: Photograph by Joanne Taylor.

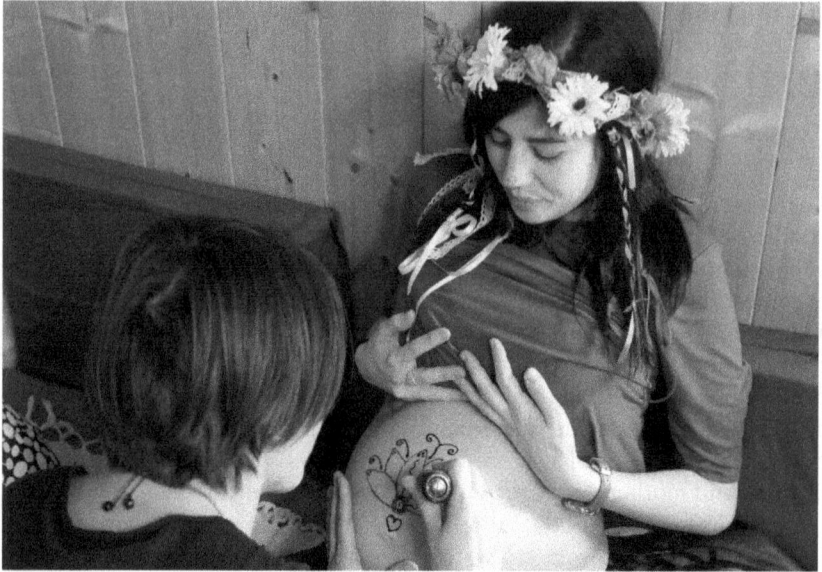

Figure 4.2 During the Blessingway, the doula is drawing on mom's belly with henna.
Source: Photograph by Joanne Taylor.

future mother considers significant to feel supported during labor and postpartum—if not physically, at least symbolically.

The Blessingway ends with the introduction of a ball of red yarn: each participant wraps a few rounds of yarn around her wrist and passes the ball to the next participant, who does the same until all present are joined. Then the thread between participant and participant is cut, and each one fastens the thread around her wrist with a knot, creating a small bracelet (see Figure 4.3). All participants will be symbolically tied together through this bracelet, which can be removed only after the birth of the child.

Dora, a doula, describes a Blessingway that she organized for a pregnant client, which she designed to accommodate the cultural preferences of her client and her non-"New-Agey" friends, as follows:

> … I did something very mild, not too meditative, just because they were not people used to or interested in that kind of thing. At first, I read a maternity story … to break the ice, and then each of them brought her own experience, if they were already mothers and the girl who was not yet a mother told what according to her was childbirth and motherhood. So, it was a good exchange, there were the first tears of emotion… We also had a moment of meditation with the music, in which they were quite quiet, but I kept it very short precisely because they were not used

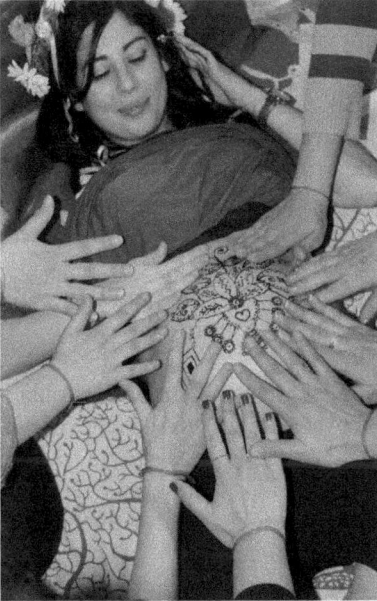

Figure 4.3 At the end of the Blessingway, all participants are tied together with a red bracelet, forming a circle of protection for the mother and baby and sending them gentle and encouraging thoughts.

Source: Photograph by Valentina Vecchiato.

[to doing this sort of thing] … As a moment of cuddling to the mother and ornament for the mother, we first built a crown with flowers … and then as an ornament…we put on nail polish, so we gave the manicure to the mother and then we all put on the nail polish, it was a very neutral thing that allowed everyone to be at ease, because henna or something a little more alternative would not be suitable… It was a nice hour of female sharing, of nonsense, a bit of little girls with the lightness that was needed for the mother and that was also needed for them to find themselves in a common dimension…

And the other wonderful moment, in my opinion, was that of the letters to the baby—each friend wrote a welcome letter to the baby and gave a gift to the mother for the post-partum. They came up with wonderful ideas…. A friend gave her an ice cream coupon, so she had 10 euros paid in the ice cream shop and when she wanted, she could go for a free ice cream. Another one gave her a breakfast coupon, and so for a month she would bring her cake or cookies for breakfast… And the third friend brought her a gift certificate, I mean "I'm going shopping for you for as long as you need and then we will go together, but in the meantime if you need things, I'll go and get them" ... You saw the commitment of people to find something useful and without spending money, in the sense of something very ... of help in the daily life for the mother in the puerperium.

We ended with the wristband, so each one greeted the others and thanked the others and tied to her wrist a red wristband that would untie only at the time of childbirth and...I asked each of them to bring a pendant and then we made her a friendship bracelet...each had a pendant and since they had known each other for a long time, each had found a pendant that was very representative of their relationship. In the end Mom realized how many people love her and this is a lot of oxytocin, in the sense that I think it filled her heart.

Since the Blessingway is an event organized for her client, if the doula is the organizer, she must be flexible and adapt the contents to the worldviews and cultural understandings of the participants, as Dora was careful to do. Dora understood that drawing with henna and long meditation were far from the systems of sensemaking recognized by participants; for this reason, she chose to offer the manicure and the nail polish instead.

Reflecting on why the Blessingway is included in doula training programs leads us to two considerations. First, bringing together the women closest to the future mother a few weeks before childbirth aims to consolidate the network of people who will be asked for support in the days to come. The absence in Italy of a real social policy to support the family after birth (Saraceno 2003) has traditionally been offset by family solidarity. The Blessingway fits into this tradition and is the occasion where requests for support are tacitly or explicitly formalized. The commitment of participants manifests through statements, gifts, and demonstrations of love. The second reflection leads us to consider the Blessingway as a ritual of preparation for childbirth. Davis-Floyd (2003, 2022), describing childbirth as a rite of passage, illustrates how this event generates a liminal/transitional experience in women between two dimensions: separation from their former identity and reintegration into their new identity as a mother. It is in this space in-between that, according to Davis-Floyd, women can experience profound inner change. Therefore, the Blessingway can also be considered a ritual of protection (Ranisio 1998) and accompaniment, supported by significative objects that give materiality to the symbolic support assured to the pregnant woman by her network of friends.

Baby showers, long common in the U.S.A., are developing in Italy. The baby shower consists of a party, usually organized by friends of the mother-to-be, to celebrate the pregnancy and give gifts to the child who will arrive and to his/her parents. The Blessingway and the baby shower differ in many aspects. First, they have different organizers: doulas organize the Blessingway, while the baby shower is generally organized by friends, and the doula is not usually invited, as she is not a friend *per se*, but rather a professional hired for a specific purpose. Secondly, the baby shower has a format that I could define as standard: it is a party designed specifically for gift-giving, while in the Blessingway, the format is individualized and customized according to the personality, tastes, and desires of the mother. Finally, the meaning attributed to the two events is different, although they share the similarity of expressing love and caring. In the baby shower, the atmosphere is lighter, while the Blessingway can bring forth deeper emotions and usually involves elements of spirituality. The Blessingway is designed to provide moments of deep self-reflection for the becoming mother, and an opportunity for the doula to invite the mother to share in the doula's holistic, spiritual ideology for a time, while the baby shower is more about just having fun. Elements of the baby shower that can carry deeper meanings include the types of gifts given: for example, a plastic baby carrier can index the likelihood of mother–baby separation at times, while a cloth baby wrap can suggest the importance of physical closeness (Davis-Floyd 2003, 2022).

Techniques and practices: relaxation and tension release

One element of the techniques and practices that unites the training programs of the three schools is represented by the techniques of contact, relaxation, and massage aimed at promoting relaxation during pregnancy and labor. For the doula, it is essential to learn to accompany the woman in the release of physical tensions and/or worries, to give her a sense of wellness in place of the sense of illness and potential pathology that dominates in technocratic births. Mondo Doula also provides a specific focus on comedy therapy—a discipline that originated in the circus and in street theater; its goal is to generate well-being through laughter. The therapeutic power of laughter has been studied since the 1980s through the development of a research field called psychoneuroendocrinoimmunology (PNEI), which has substantiated a direct correlation between the psyche and the nervous, endocrine, and immune systems (see Pert 1997).

Techniques and practices: accompaniment, support, and art counseling

Other aspects of the techniques and practices that unite the trainings of Mondo Doula and Mammadoula are related to accompaniment and support in labor, and the tools to deal with simple problems in the pregnancy and postpartum period. The doula interlocutors learned how to give massages and how to help the laboring woman change positions to alleviate the pain. In addition, the doula must know how to set up the context for labor: provide soft lights; background music if the woman wishes; offer food, drinks, blankets, hot water bags, fans, and in general anything that can bring comfort in those moments. Even in cases of hospital labor, the doula has the task of paying attention to these aspects to make the experience of childbirth as nonviolent and gentle as possible (Leboyer 1974). As part of their tool kit for dealing with physiological discomforts, the doulas are taught to suggest natural infusions to relieve nausea during pregnancy, or, in the last weeks of gestation, to support women to look for comfortable positions or pillow arrangements to ensure a more pleasant rest. In cases of difficulties in breastfeeding, doulas provide simple suggestions and, if the situation does not improve, they advise the mother to contact the midwife or the breastfeeding expert available in the area.

This part of the training is also closely linked to the development of relational skills. Much time is dedicated by all three schools to the care of the mother, the newborn, and the presence of the doula within the family. Taking care of household chores and other children, preparing meals, running errands, managing visits of relatives and friends, proposing walks and moments of leisure are all actions that the students must learn and practice to support the new mother.

Mondo Doula is the only school that has introduced into its training a module on art counseling. Art counseling is a discipline based on therapeutic counseling, which is implemented using artistic forms: dance, music, theater, painting, sculpture, and other artistic languages. Through the artistic form, the doula aims to bring out emotions that can generate tensions and can affect the client's well-being. Motherhood brings with it a creative potential, a feminine force analogous to the loving pleasure that gives life and shapes the embryo, but the prevalence of scientific rationality has silenced these ways of knowing, to the point where the technocratic model has appropriated and defused the vitality not only of the placenta but also of the maternal body (Vegetti Finzi 1990). In contrast to the technocratic model, doulas use the tools of art to unleash maternal creativity, recognizing its expressive potential, which, they feel, has never been sufficiently exalted.

Techniques and practices: placenta rituals and birthstory narration

From the narratives of doulas emerges the choice by those women who opt for lotus birth to celebrate the placenta through a ritual that in some cases they help to realize. Once cord separation has occurred, some women choose to bury the placenta in their home garden, sometimes planting a tree near or on top of the place where they buried it; others freeze it and plant it later on, also organizing a party of celebration. Some mothers eat the placenta or send it to specialized companies in Germany or the United Kingdom (since in Italy it is forbidden by law to deal with this preparation) to be transformed into pills and used as a supplement, so that they can benefit from the hormones and nutrients contained in it to prevent postpartum depression and in general to reduce pain. Some data on the perceptions and experiences of women who have chosen placentophagy indicate a considerable benefit in terms of postnatal health; however, a literature review carried out by some US researchers (Coyle et al. 2015) does not confirm a real benefit attributable to this practice. If in some animal species placentophagy has some positive outcomes, these outcomes do not appear to extend to humans, and data in this sense have not yet been produced. But no matter what science says, if a woman wishes to practice a lotus birth or celebrate the placenta or any other related practice or ritual, the doula will do her utmost to facilitate its realization.

The narration of the birth story is a process through which the doula proposes to the mother to tell the entire story of her path from pregnancy to childbirth. This technique aims to retrace the experience in a reflective way; the doula guides the client through the story and solicits insights, emphasizing memories and positive feelings and emotions, trying to lighten any negative ones. According to Davis-Floyd (personal correspondence, August 2021), "stories give meaning and coherence to experience," thereby helping the new mother to come to terms with her birth experience and to integrate its meaning—and perhaps alter that meaning in a positive way if needed. The doula will also take care of writing what is narrated to set it in memory in a tangible way.

Techniques and practices: peer groups, mothers' circles, and the Red Tent

Mammadoula is the only school that has chosen to introduce a module on peer groups and the Red Tent. Training on peer groups aims to provide the tools for managing groups, since some of the activities that doulas offer are trainings for pregnant mothers or pregnant couples, and mother's circles:

> Mother's circles are free meetings ... they are held once every two weeks ... usually there is always me or another doula of the association and then a colleague that deals with child massage. Mothers come with children, from pregnancy up to 15 months, who know us through the internet, Facebook, or flyers. We propose a theme, which is usually not respected because the goal is to meet mothers and allow them to relax, chat, be with other women... Starting to make mother's circles was a good start to spread, to make known the figure of the doula in this city, because it is not known at all.
>
> (Lisa)

Such meetings aim to generate sharing and support among women who are living similar experiences and, at the same time, act as promotional opportunities for doulas, because they have the possibility to make themselves known and to engage potential clients.

Mammadoula incorporates a module on the "Red Tent," which consists of an opportunity to meet women of any age, to reflect, compare, and share thoughts and emotions. The book *The Red Tent* by Anita Diamant, published in 1997, has inspired many women internationally. The story rewrites part of *Genesis* and is narrated in the first person by Dinah, the last child and only daughter of Jacob. The author develops the story by taking inspiration from the biblical story of Dinah, her mother Leah, and the other wives of Jacob to imagine their everyday lives, which develop, despite the tensions, through different roles and functions via the creation of a kind of matriarchal village separated from the lives of men. The Red Tent is the place where women gather in important moments: where they retire on menstruation days, where they celebrate every new moon, where they spend their pregnancies and give birth to their children. Through this text, the author offers an interpretation of a patriarchal religion from a female and feminist point of view (Blackford 2005). Following the tradition of the Red Tent as narrated by Diamant, some doulas interviewed decided to implement this practice, considering these meetings necessary so women can share experiences related to female cyclicality and confronting difficulties or doubts. The Red Tent is usually organized once a month and the spaces that host it are decorated with red carpets and curtains; the participants sit on the ground creating a circle. The facilitators propose a theme or a reflection, and the group members interact, respecting the opinions or choices of others. Participants are also asked not to judge and to keep secret everything said. The Red Tent celebrates female cyclicity and honors the need for space and time for sharing, allowing women to devote time to reflection and introspection. Including the Red Tent in the training program provides students with tools to organize and conduct meetings and rituals and, at the same time, implies the will to promote a "new" practice that allows groups of women to meet and share everyday life in a space that feels both sacred and safe. (For descriptions of "Pink" and "Ruby" Tents in the U.S.A. for young girls and teenagers, see Davis-Floyd and Laughlin 2022.)

Communication elements

The communication elements refer to techniques that students must learn to communicate effectively with their clients. In all three programs, this dimension receives a deep focus, yet only Mondo Doula pays attention to interactions with healthcare professionals. In the narratives of interlocutors, this communicative aspect is described as the ability to accurately choose the vocabulary to use, the most appropriate tone of voice and the gestures to adopt to create an appropriate and receptive style of interaction that keeps the focus on the client and makes her feel comfortable, listened to, and safe.

The social context and professional networking: mapping facilities and services

Another area in the practical skills is the social context and professional network. All three trainings provide tools that enable students to map the services aimed at pregnant and postpartum women in the area where they live. This includes knowing the facilities where women can give birth and their protocols, making contacts and starting collaborations with other professionals (gynecologists, pediatricians, midwives, IBCLCs, osteopaths, etc.), getting to know the associations that offer services, activities, and paths for pregnant women and new mothers, and finally to always keep up-to-date on meetings, conferences, and workshops that may interest the client.

The social context and professional networking: support for returning to work

Mondo Doula and Mammadoula also consider it essential to provide students with tools to fit into any family context, to be aware of the special characteristics unique to each family. It is also essential to encourage the creation of family and friend networks to support the mother. Mondo Doula also explores the themes of motherhood and work. The doulas interviewed say that returning to work is generally difficult for new mothers, both because of the separation from the newborn and the need to continue to manage everyday family affairs. The doula must therefore be able to support the woman in this passage, proposing concrete solutions to the difficulties that arise.

Marketing and client relationship management

The last area of doula trainings concerns the marketing and client management elements. Only Mondo Doula and Mammadoula offer training in this field; this allows us to imagine not only the will to equip students with tools suitable to manage their professional activities but also underlies the vision that these two associations have of the doula: a professional capable of self-promoting, finding the most suitable communication channels, and being able to maintain a rewarding relationship with the client. The management of the doula–client relationship seems particularly delicate: the doula's frequent visits to her clients' homes and the co-creation of a confidential and intimate relationship could make this relationship assume the traits of friendship, compromising the professional character of the service and potentially making it more difficult for the mother to let go of this relationship when the time comes. For this reason, it is essential to equip students with tools to prevent this risk; as Nora described,

> Usually in the moment of knowledge, I propose a contract to the mother that I noticed can give security to me, but also to the mother to have me … I have found this double side … a contract that says what I can do, what I cannot do, and what I must not do.

This contract is one of the tools used to offer a guarantee of seriousness and professionalism, but also to clarify the professional limits of competence, given the ongoing widespread lack of knowledge in Italy about the doula and her roles. Helping the client to define her needs and desires, deciding the times and methods of support, as well as identifying the time when the doula's role with that particular client will end, appear to be fundamental skills for the doula.

Students must also acquire tools to promote themselves and to spread the knowledge of the doula profile. Competence assessment or SWOT analysis (a strategic planning technique used to identify Strengths, Weaknesses, Opportunities, and Threats related to business activities) is necessary to define the professional project and to adapt it according to the objectives set. The students are also trained to identify the most appropriate advertising channels for their objectives and needs. In relation to this aspect, doulas' stories highlight different experiences: some doulas believe in the potential of the Internet and have created their own website, social network page, or blog, where they write reflections and share experiences and photographs that represent them and the services they provide. Others say they are not very familiar with the Internet and prefer to create leaflets to leave in shops and associations frequented by mothers, or to organize meetings, book presentations, and conferences. However, according to their narratives, the best advertising is the word of mouth among mothers; as Alda noted, "In my opinion the word of mouth is the best thing—it makes culture—that is if I followed the mother X then she will talk about it, and consequently the marketing strategy is there for me." The doula is a figure who frequents the client's home environment and builds an intimate and deep relationship with the client, and that is why word of mouth is the best advertisement. A positive experience of a mother, friend, or family member is a guarantee to others of the quality of service that particularly doula provides.

Relational and emotional skills

Relational skills are considered by the doulas interviewed to be the main characteristics of their profession. I have identified three areas in which these types of skills are developed: elements of analysis and assessment of needs; relational and reflective elements; and elements of psychology, anthropology, and philosophy.

The elements of analysis and assessment of needs are developed only in the trainings of Mondo Doula and Mammadoula, since they consider fundamental that the doula should understand the mother's needs, considering and evaluating the system of values that she holds. To manage this part of the work, doulas are also required to be constantly updated on the scientific literature on the perinatal period. The system of knowledge that doulas use to legitimize their assessments and considerations is constituted on the one hand by the humanistic model of assistance to pregnancy and childbirth (Davis Floyd 2001, 2018, 2022); on the other hand, the doula's model of care must merge with the client's knowledge system. The doula must therefore act and think flexibly, responding to the mother's needs in ways that respect her manner of thinking—just as the doula does in designing the Blessingway.

The relational and reflective elements group together the aspects that most characterize the doula profile. The three schools agree on some training dimensions regarding these elements; Mondo Doula dedicates greater depth to this area. All three training courses deepen the theme of "active listening" as a major way of supporting the client. Active listening requires the skill of accepting the mother's sometimes bewildering and disorienting thoughts and beliefs, wonderings, and imaginings, in order to draw from the doula toolbox possible words or solutions (Sclavi 2003); as Mina describes,

> What a doula does ... is that she doesn't stick her nose into your business... [laughs], but simply... listens to you .... she is there with you .... and this in my opinion is the special thing of our work, what there just is nowhere else.

Knowing how to listen to women without judgment, so that they can express their moods and desires freely, and eventually ask questions that may trigger a reflective process, are fundamental characteristics of a good doula. For any choice the mother and/or the couple decide to make, the doula has the task of being with them in that choice; in the case of indecision or difficulty, the doula will support the mother in exploring the range of possibilities and paths available; she will not dictate what the mother should do (Praetorius 2002). Listening takes place in the familiar environment of the client's home. One of the primary characteristics of the doula, as emerged from the interviews, is not to pose herself as an expert:

> The doula has a very soft approach, very professional but at the same time friendly, affective, home, domestic, is a reassuring figure ... One thing women complain about is when they say, "The midwife told me to do this," or "The gynecologist told me to do this," this thing about the "you have to do this", you have to, you have to, there's always someone telling you have to .... Here the doula does not do this.
>
> (Alba)

The creation of a friendly relationship emerges from interlocutors' stories as indispensable to developing a deep contact with the woman and the family. However, the type of approach adopted assumes specific characteristics: on the one hand, the doula is far from the figure of the expert, since she does not establish a relationship confined to an exclusive disciplinary area; on the other hand, the doula must create a relationship with her client that is somewhat distanced from family or friends and that is also nonjudgmental. Relatives and friends may judge; doulas do not. The doula must know how to be close to women and families, be there for them, stand by, and listen actively, and these requirements cannot be learned through techniques but must be experienced and become incorporated attitudes. These elements merge in a confidential, nonmanagerial professional style, which differs both from the styles of the healthcare professionals and of family members, highlighting the construction of a new professional field where places and modes of interaction differ from those of existing models.

A further element that characterizes the profile of the doula and that is present in the three training programs refers to what Mondo Doula and Mammadoula define as empowerment, while Progetto Primo Respiro speaks of maieutics (in Italian, *maieutica*), which refers to the Socratic method of eliciting knowledge by a series of questions and answers; as Emma explains, "try to help the mother find her own resources and answers." Following Mosedale (2005), there are four aspects generally recognized in the literature as constituting the concept of "empowerment." First, and paradoxically, a subject must be disempowered to be empowered. From the stories of the interlocutors, this aspect emerges in relation to the reasons why they are contacted by mothers who attribute a sense of disempowerment linked to the condition of pregnancy or maternity, the fragility of this time, and the sense of loneliness often experienced. The second aspect refers to the fact that empowerment cannot be treated as a transferable process but must be desired and needed by those who live a condition of disempowerment. The actions to be implemented to promote empowerment must facilitate a personal activation process. In the case of doulas, this process occurs from the first contact with her client. The client's request for support substantiates an activation by mothers that doulas must only welcome and encourage. The third aspect of empowerment refers to a decision-making attitude and actions regarding issues considered important by disempowered people. Reflection, analysis, and action are involved in this process, which can develop at individual or collective levels. In the representations of the doula interlocutors, this aspect emerges strongly. They described with satisfaction those actions taken by clients that subvert unhelpful family traditions, or that subvert actions on the part of healthcare professionals considered by mothers as not befitting their wishes. The fourth aspect highlights empowerment not as a result, but as a process. One never gets to be empowered in an absolute sense, but the individual and eventually collective process is defined in relation to others or in relation to oneself. This aspect is present in doulas' discourses related to the conclusion of their relationship with the client. The end of this relationship occurs in most cases because the mother has become aware of what is meaningful to her and no longer needs doula support. Nevertheless, again, it can sometimes be quite difficult for the mother to let go of her doula, especially when the client has come to rely on the doula's remarkable emotional support—which is why doulas must carefully navigate and sometime stress the professionalism of their relationships with their clients, in order to avoid this risk of dependence.

Although the main feature of the doula profile is relational, Mondo Doula is the only association that details in its training program the aspects of relationship that are deepened in doula–client interactions. Students must, for example, be able to work on confidence, building a trust-based relationship with the client; must know how to use a metaphor as a tool, so clients can express themselves and face difficulties; must become familiar with the use of poetic language to dialogue and converse drawing on new vocabulary. Doulas can propose to clients to write a poem or to read one together, or to choose among several poems which one best reflects the client's emotions. The goal of using poems or songs is to explore emotions, allowing fears or doubts or happiness to find a channel of expression. These aspects of the training course contribute to characterizing the professional field of doulas. Mondo Doula also dedicates a specific focus to fathers/partners:

> even men were not born fathers as women were not born mothers … They often feel lost too, suddenly find themselves with a whole series of responsibilities that maybe they did not expect… then the presence of the doula in the family dynamic can be important.
>
> (Rita)

Doulas have also the task of supporting fathers/partners in the rite of passage of the birth and in the new family's process of adaptation. Considering the specific needs and fears of fathers/partners is necessary for the well-being of the whole family. The meanings can be manifold: supporting the husband/partner can for example consolidate the confidence that the woman places in the doula or, since often it is the husband/partner who is in charge of the economic support of the family, it may serve to make him/her appreciate the doula for whose services he is paying. And dealing with fathers/partners can foster the deconstruction of traditional representations of masculinity and paternity.

Additionally, Mondo Doula deepens the aspect of meditation and centering of the doula. Like other caring professions, the doula has the task of acting as a "mirror" for the mother; the doula must be "centered" to avoid projecting her own traumas and emotions onto the client. Meditation can be a tool that supports doulas to find centering; in this way they can support mothers. To be able to take care of other people, doulas must first deal with themselves, must seek and answer the question: "Who am I really?" It is only through self-recognition that recognition in relationships is possible (Bertolo 2013).

The last area of relational competence concerns the elements of psychology and philosophy. In this sector, Mondo Doula and Progetto Primo Respiro offer a wide range of trainings, while Mammadoula seems to be more limited. All three training courses deepen the psychological dimension related to motherhood and its potential for personal growth and evolution. Becoming a mother can generate tensions and difficulties but, at the same time, can open up new possibilities. The students must learn to grasp the profound transformations that can take place in the client, and the representations and meanings linked to the experience of motherhood, in order to accompany her on this path. Mondo Doula pays close attention to this area by addressing numerous features related to the experience of becoming a mother: fears, prejudices, pain, anger, frustration, fatigue, the spiritual aspects of becoming a mother, and anxieties about potential difficulties in childbirth. Progetto Primo Respiro instead focuses more on the transformations that the birth can bring within the couple, and on the configurations that could characterize the new family.

All three training courses include the baby blues in their trainings, while Mondo Doula and Progetto Primo Respiro make it clear that they also deal with depression through their trainers, who are psychologists. The absence in the Mammadoula program of a deepening of the learning about postpartum depression seems dictated by the desire to respect the boundaries of professional competence: depression is within the competence of the psychologist or psychiatrist. However, the importance attached by all three associations to this aspect is clear: the doula must be able to detect the typical signals of the baby blues and must intervene promptly to get this mother whatever kind of help she needs to prevent the baby blues from turning into full-scale postpartum depression.

Considering the development of the relational skills that characterize doula practice, and the need to be flexible and adapt the approach to the client, I can affirm that in this profession, the dimension of the immateriality of doula work is crucial (La Rosa 2005; Maestripieri 2013). This aspect is evident through the strong relational component of doula care, which is based on impalpable bonds of trust.

Doulas' training methodologies

The training methodologies that characterize the three paths analyzed and reflected in the doulas' professional methods and styles appear very homogeneous. One element that emerges as fundamental concerns the elaboration of the personal experience. As previously noted, any traumatic experiences that each student has lived through need to be investigated and analyzed to avoid transferring personal problems to the client; in psychology, this is called "projection." Experiential knowledge, as theorized by Jedlowski (1986), differs from scientific knowledge and that of "common sense," because it finds nourishment from daily life, doubting and questioning its meaning. What the students must therefore learn is a process of permanent auto-reflexivity (Piazza 2013)—a construction of their biographies based on a daily attitude of self-questioning. Each school uses its own method to develop this process: Mondo Doula and Mammadoula utilize group supervision and storytelling, while Progetto Primo Respiro does not explicate the method used. Nina, who was trained by Mondo Doula, explains,

> ... active listening was the strongest work we have done in groups or in pairs, so standing in front of a future colleague who cries, without

touching her, without interrupting the emotions, this was in my opinion the [most] important work that has been done in my training.

Talking about their personal experiences within the school helps students to develop competence in active listening and to incorporate the communicative styles to be adopted in interactions with clients. These include awareness of the importance and meanings of gestures, facial mimicry, and bodily postures. The incorporation of professional practices and helpful communicative styles can also take place through role playing, more commonly called *simulata* (simulation). The simulata aims to stage a situation typical of the doulas' repertoire. The trainer defines the script, which usually involves a mother with a specific need and a doula, and the students are invited to role-play the different actors, with the aim of learning to find balance and thereby to benefit the mother or family. At the end of the simulation, the same trainer takes on the role of expert doula, highlighting the positive and negative aspects of the interactions. Through this role-playing, students learn to face situations that can occur in the working context, in this "do in the moment" situation. Even though it is a simulation, it still provides the opportunity to internalize an embodied practical knowledge that forges the constitution of a lasting repertoire of practices (Bruni and Gherardi 2007). Additionally, Mondo Doula and Mammadoula provide the presence of a tutor, also called "godmother," who will accompany the students throughout their training, serving as a point of reference and introducing them to the doula community during their training or after its completion.

The basic course is a first step in doula training and aims to teach the most essential skills; however, interviews with professional doulas have revealed many similar paths followed in parallel or later, with the aim of broadening their knowledge and continuing the work on themselves begun during their initial training. The paths are extremely heterogeneous; below is a brief description of the main ongoing trainings mentioned:

* **Babywearing:** Different associations offer trainings to become "babywearing consultants."[1] Many doulas attend this training because the wrap is a useful tool for mothers as it favors contact, helps to strengthen the mother–child or father–child relationship, and generally nurtures the newborn.
* **Breastfeeding:** Breastfeeding can be difficult for new mothers, and breastfeeding support is one of the more common requests doulas encounter. For this reason, it seems important, from the stories of interlocutors, to have knowledge about the physiology of breastfeeding. Generally, the training courses mentioned refer to the WHO–UNICEF[2]

1 http://scuoladelportare.it/; www.portareipiccoli.org/; www.mammacanguro.com/.
2 www.who.int/maternal_child_adolescent/documents/pdfs/bc_trainers_guide.pdf.

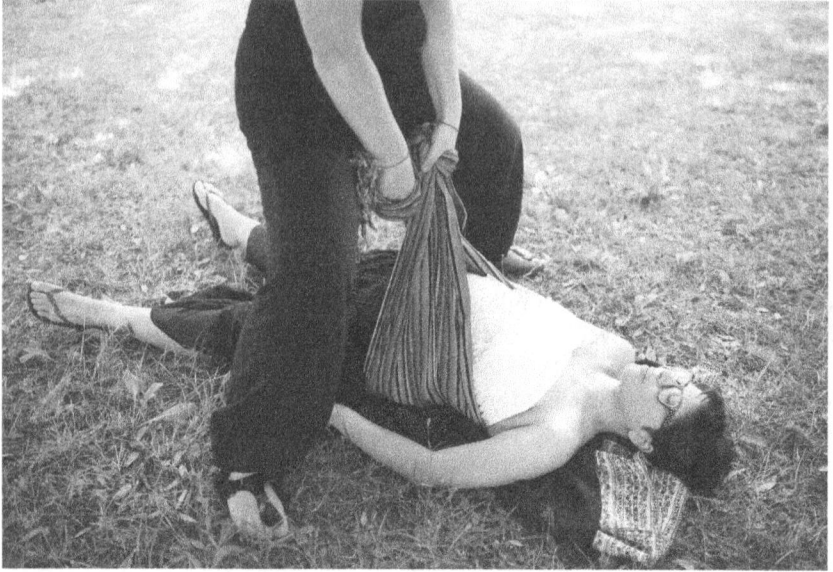

Figure 4.4 A doula practicing massage with a rebozo.
Source: Photograph by Valentina Dalla Pria.

model or to the path to becoming an IBCLC (International Board-Certified Lactation Consultant).[3]

- **Massage:** The training courses followed by doulas in relation to massage techniques are divided into two strands: massages to be taught to parents to use on their newborns; and massages to be practiced on women to relieve tensions and alleviate pain. In the first group were mentioned the trainings offered by AIMI (Italian Association for Child Massage)[4] and by the Italian Association for Child Massage Shantala[5]; in the second group are the techniques of massage with a *rebozo*,[6] (as shows Figure 4.4) and/or bioenergetic massage.
- **Movement:** Doulas narrate that movement and dance are useful tools to relieve stress and tensions in pregnant women and, in particular, refer to the training offered by MIPA (International Active Childbirth Movement)

3 http://iblce.org/.
4 www.aimionline.it/.
5 www.massaggioinfantileshantala.it/.
6 A shawl of Mexican origin traditionally used in childbirth for massage or for repositioning the baby in utero, or as a wrap to carry babies. In Italy, there is not yet an organization that deals exclusively with this type of training; usually the trainers are hosted by different associations. The trainers mentioned by interlocutors, who held rebozo courses in Italy, come from the Netherlands. http://rebozo.nl/indexe.html.

on movement and the perineum in pregnancy and postpartum,[7] to the Rio Abierto method,[8] to *biodanza*,[9] and to emotional and body work.[10]

- **Singing:** The potentials of singing to relieve pain during labor and childbirth, and in general to give expression to emotions, have led some doulas to choose to deepen their knowledge of how to use song. The paths refer to the technique of carnatic singing[11] and techniques of psychophony[12] and audio analgesia.[13]

- **Harmonization of scars:** This is an osteopathic technique, taught by David Kanner, to be practiced on women who have had a cesarean birth. Some doulas choose to undertake this training to support mothers who had a cesarean and were traumatized by the experience. The goal of the technique is to restore harmony and balance to the scar and in general to the whole body.

- **Perinatal mourning:** The choice to deepen this theme emerges in the stories of interlocutors, because it is considered important to support mothers who live the experience of an abortion, whether spontaneous, elective, or therapeutic, or who experience a fetal or newborn death. The training courses mentioned refer to the courses offered by the association "Ciao Lapo"[14] and the annual conference of the association Iris (Research Institute for Health Intervention).[15]

- **Education:** Many doulas choose to become perinatal educators through a course offered by the International Movement for Active Childbirth (MIPA), or prenatal and neonatal educators through a course offered by the University of Padua,[16] or other courses offered by ANEP (National Association of Professional Educators).[17]

- **Active listening/Counseling:** some doulas have chosen to undertake courses to learn counseling techniques or to improve their ability to listen actively.

  Paths "to the feminine": An area of interest for some doulas consists of those paths that the interlocutors define as "feminine" and include insights on female cyclicality, such as the path to becoming a "moon mother"[18] or to manage the lunar and menstrual calendar.

---

7 www.mipaonline.com/.
8 www.rioabiertoitalia.org/.
9 www.biodanza.it/.
10 www.willi-maurer.ch/.
11 Carnatic singing is a chant native to India that has been popularized in Europe since the 1970s by the French obstetrician Frédérick Leboyer.
12 This is a holistic approach to singing based on body awareness. It was created and developed by Marie-Louise Aucher in the early 1960s. The main goal of psychophonie is to deepen a person's experience as a whole integrated being.
13 https://seaoscuola.it/.
14 www.ciaolapo.it/.
15 www.irisassociazione.it/.
16 www.unipd.it/corso-perfezionamento-educatore-prenatale-neonatale.
17 www.anep.it/.
18 www.wombblessing.com.

Rituals and relational models

The participant observation that I carried out in a training course and in seminars and workshops for doulas allowed me to grasp some dimensions characterizing the definition of the doula through practices that embody models of interaction and relationship:

> We sit in the space that had been prepared, sitting in a circle on cushions with a candle in the middle and some dried fruit…The facilitators start, introduce the workshop, and ask that each of us, after presenting ourselves in the way she prefers, say three things about herself: two true and one false, and the group will have to identify the lie. So, one by one we introduce ourselves. The circle is a moment in which each is free to present herself as she wishes and to say what she wants. The little game of saying two true things and a false one is cute and allows you to know something more about us.
>
> (Diary notes from Mimosa festival)

> At 9 there is the appointment in the room where the seminar will be held for the opening circle. Slowly we sit in a circle and there are always children running back and forth, the organizer takes the floor and welcomes us. Then she asks us to make a presentation tour by saying our name and a word that represents us in this seminar. Various words come out, the most recurrent are trust, love, deepening, sisterhood, curiosity, research, emotions, welcome.
>
> (Diary notes from Primrose festival)

> Participants take off their shoes and sit down on the ground, where colored cushions are placed in a circle. The hosts introduce the event, and it is proposed [to participants] to present themselves through a game: the game of "If I Were". Each participant has to say what a doula is through this game and the question is "If you were a movie, what movie would you be?" The tour begins and numerous films are mentioned: "Fried green tomatoes"; "Antonia"; "Ehrengard"; "The green planet"; "Amour"; "*Io sono con te*" ("I am with you"); "Women on the verge of a nervous breakdown." Leda says "Avatar" because the doula aspires high like those blue guys. Mina says "Bagdad cafè," because right now she feels a little lost in the work she's doing. Ines says "The house of the spirits," because there is a child who becomes a woman and there is a wisdom that is handed down among women through love, magic, life beyond death. Ines adds "The meaning of life" by Monty Python because it perfectly describes the horrors of the hospital. Finally, Bice mentions "Ponyo," as it is the only cartoon in which a woman is seen breastfeeding. Cleo takes the floor and says, "Like water for chocolate" because the magic ingredient is love, and then two other movies that came to her are "A walk in the clouds," as she remembers the scene where women sew together, creating

a circle who share chatter and create a unique thing (the quilt) and says that this is typical of doulas, working together to create a unique thing.

(Diary notes from Hortensia festival)

An element present in all doulas' meetings consists in sitting on the ground arranged in a circle. The circularity aims to enshrine equality among those present. Like the trainers or facilitators of the event, each participant is invited to speak freely, sharing thoughts and reflections to enrich the conversation. The equality offered by the circularity, however, does not translate into fungibility. The role of leading or moderating always remains in the hands of the trainer or the event organizer. Although there are no elements that materially denote the difference in status, deference to the moderator is noticeable; usually doulas speak without contradicting, out of respect and admiration for the trainers.

Another feature of doulas' meetings is the way they are presented. The request of the facilitators to tell something about themselves, sometimes by citing a film or choosing a word, refers to dimensions related to the life experiences of each participant. Their differing backgrounds appear irrelevant in this doula training; through images, metaphors, and poetic words, doulas describe their own experiences, communicate with others (Siebert 2012), and prepare themselves to welcome new ideas. Experiential knowledge deeply informs the training and the activities of the doulas. Taking part in such seminars and workshops demonstrates doulas' or doula students' implicit willingness to join in a ritual of self-disclosure, of sharing one's own experiences, which is facilitated by the circular formation that conveys the principle of equality between participants:

> … at this point the trainer proposes a new workshop. She divides the students into pairs. In turn one is invited to play the mother and the other the fetus, and then the roles are reversed. Fetuses lie down and close their eyes. Music is played that reproduces the heartbeat and then there are relaxing songs. The trainer put in the center of the room cotton balls soaked in essential oils, other foods, and spices (salt, chili, sugar, coffee, cinnamon), small musical instruments (rattles, tambourines, castanets, maracas), and a bottle of water. Each couple focuses on the workshop: the one who plays the mother cuddles the fetus, caresses her, stimulates her with musical instruments, makes her smell the scents, taste the flavors, and then when they consider the experience completed, without speaking, they invert the roles. In the end, the trainer invites the students to exchange impressions, first in pairs and then with the group. The aim of the workshop is to understand the wide sensory capacities of the fetus during pregnancy. Children in utero have sensory experiences, hear noises, feel tastes, and perceive contact, and sensory channels are a system of communication with the child. What the mother eats gladly is a message of pleasure for the child.

(Diary notes from Rose festival)

When we are all ready, the trainers proposed a massage session. A group does and a group receives and then the roles are reversed. We sit on the ground in the lounge area, dim the lights and put on some "New Age" music, massage the feet of the companion, about 15 minutes per foot. The technique of massage is often used by doulas, both to offer to the mothers and between doulas to take care of and to pamper each other. After the massage, the exchange of a hug or a kiss takes place in almost all couples.

(Diary notes from Mimosa festival)

The workshops, role-playing games, and massages implemented during trainings are intended to stimulate the learning of the relationship models that characterize the doula profession. Taking care of one's colleagues and companions, as shows Figure 4.5, and embodying these rituals of care are necessary and functional for the performance of the professional activity.

The attention to the context, the choice of music, and possibly the objects to use are integral parts of the training, which aims to stimulate

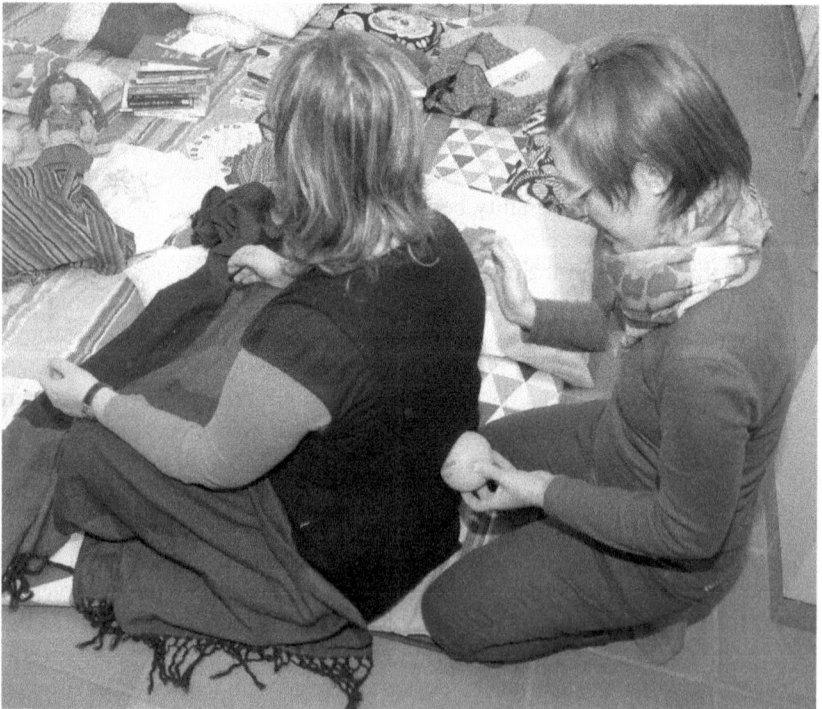

Figure 4.5 Doulas taking care of each other. A doula practicing a gentle back massage on a colleague.
Source: Photograph by Licia Valso.

the doula's ability to explore multiple ways and forms of caregiving. The doula must be able to merge knowledge with experience and to implement this know-how through relational models and practices of care that are lived and embodied. Knowledge and practice—the spheres of intimacy and professional life—appear to feed each other and give life to a professional profile that encompasses the diversities of women's lifeworlds and emotions.

Conclusion

My analysis of the training paths to becoming a doula in Italy reveals a profile that is difficult to define, as each doula school seems to define it differently. I did find homogeneity in the training of relational skills, the models of relationship, and in the methodologies used to shape the professional style of the doula. However, some aspects of the training courses differ among schools, and the heterogeneity of extra trainings shows an extremely dynamic profile, constantly evolving, that rejects a crystallized definition of knowledge and skills.

The system of knowledge to which the doula refers is therefore pluralistic. It's not only one knowledge system, but many. At first analysis, the cultural base on which the activity is anchored might appear incoherent, fragile, and destined not to support the development of the doula profile. Yet at a level of deeper reflection, we can observe a coherence that I characterize as "patchwork" (Balbo 2008)—as in the creation of the abovementioned quilt. Starting with practices, the trainings integrate cultural elements. In other words, doula practices give coherence to the pluralism of symbols and systems of knowledge to which the doulas refer and which they incorporate. It is in the patchwork, in the ability to assimilate different and coexisting knowledge systems, that the doula fashions her own patterns of meaning. The need for continuous evolution appears to be an essential condition for doulas, both to continue self-reflexivity and the introspective work begun within the basic training, and to constantly continue to equip themselves with new tools to support women and families. The change and expansion of her cultural base is therefore a constant condition of the profile of the doula and becomes one of the essential characteristics of her professionalism (Barley and Kunda 2004; Vicarelli 2012; Maestripieri 2013).

5   The doula profession

The analysis of a profession needs to be conducted via the work that constitutes that profession. Investigating, through doulas' narratives, the contexts, activities, and aspects considered essential in the performance of the doula's work is fundamental for understanding the ways in which claims for specific arenas of jurisdiction are made. As shown in Chapter 3, the links between work and jurisdictions determine the social control of the profession.

Doulas' work

In my analyses of the training paths necessary to become a doula in Italy (Chapter 4), I outlined the characteristics of the doula; here, I will explicate the characteristics of doula practice and note that the reasons for competition with other professions lie in the actions that characterize the work itself (Abbott 1988). The interlocutors explained that their first contact with potential clients takes place by phone, e-mail, or Facebook. During this first interaction with the client (and/or with her partner), the doula listens to the client's needs, explains her skills, and sets up a face-to-face meeting. During this first meeting, which usually takes place at the client's home, the doula further explores the needs of the mother-to-be, proposes support strategies, and states her fee. What is agreed orally is sometimes written down in a contract, which is signed during the following meeting. Other doulas consider a verbal agreement to be sufficient, since the relationship is built on mutual trust. Some doulas leave this decision up to the mother; as Tina said, "there are some women who need the contract and I do it, other women who would be scared with the contract and I don't." The flexibility of the doula in understanding the needs of the client and adapting to them is therefore crucial even during the definition of the employment relationship. Once the type of support required is clarified, the doula begins her work with that client.

DOI: 10.4324/9781003165934-6

Pregnancy

During pregnancy, doula work consists of multiple types of actions: accompanying the client to her prenatal appointments; helping her with errands and domestic chores; encouraging her to write a birth plan and helping her to construct it, if she wishes; accompanying her to visit the facilities where she can give birth or helping her to find a midwife for childbirth at home; listening to her and encouraging her to express her fears surrounding pregnancy and birth; supporting her to elaborate on any traumatic experiences she may have had, including trauma from prior births; suggesting the practice of relaxation techniques or visualizations that may help during labor, as shows Figure 5.1; encouraging her to express her creativity through writing, painting, dancing, etc., as shows Figure 5.2; proposing outings or walks; organizing the Blessingway (see Chapter 4); and in general taking care of everything the client may need:

> ... we get ready for the event, see videos together, do some visualization exercises, prepare the baby's room, go to choose the baby wrap or other tools that might be useful ...

> (Elga)

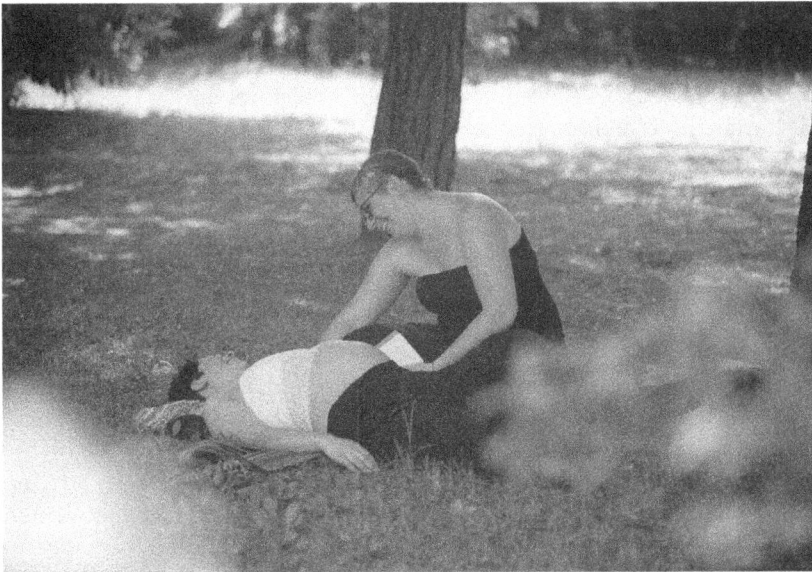

Figure 5.1 A doula proposing a relaxation and visualization to the pregnant mother. Source: Photograph by Valentina Dalla Pria.

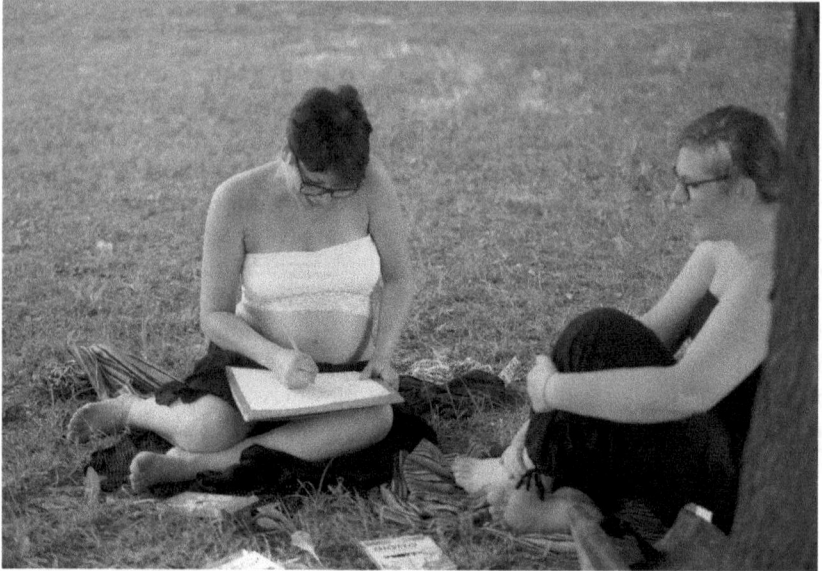

Figure 5.2 A doula invites the pregnant mother to express her thoughts and wishes through drawing.

Source: Photograph by Valentina Dalla Pria.

> With my last client, we did some singing meetings during pregnancy—for me this is an important tool to get in touch with the woman and for her to get in contact with the child. We met several times and she asked me to accompany her to her check-ups. She needed to talk and I noticed that the singing moment helped to create the right atmosphere to allow her to open herself up to the relationship with me.
>
> (Clio)

Some doulas, generally in collaboration with other professionals (midwife, counselor, psychologist, child masseuse), choose to create paths for women or couples to follow during pregnancy and birth. These paths are not proposed in an alternative way to those provided by the hospital or the health department, but rather with the aim of offering a space to reflect on needs, emotions, hopes, and dreams of the woman and her partner. Other doulas, after specific training, offer trainings in yoga or dance during the pregnancy, and in "sweet gymnastics"—a kind of gymnastics in which you avoid heavy exercises that could overstrain a body already engaged in such a delicate task. Others work on voice, breath, and singing as tools to be used in labor to channel and release pain.

Labor and birth

> ... when I attend births, which happens very rarely... be there, be by the side, motivate, encourage ... this is what I do.

> (Rosa)

Doula's support during labor and childbirth emerges from the stories of the interlocutors as happening sporadically, both because the doula profile is not yet well known in Italy and because it is generally the partner who supports the woman, since almost all Italian hospitals allow only one labor companion. The reasons why women ask for doula assistance are often linked to a desire to replace the partner if he/she doesn't want to assist or is not available, or if the mother doesn't want the partner to be with her during labor and birth, or in cases of single mothers. The doula can also be preferred to a relative or friend, thanks to the relationship of trust that she can establish with her client and to her non-involvement in family or friendship dynamics. Doulas who accompany women during labor and birth generally offer 24/7 availability, starting two weeks before the due date. During labor, doula practices consist of relaxation techniques; lessening pain with simple massages, sometimes through the use of the rebozo (Italian doulas don't practice the baby repositioning technique for which the rebozo can also be used, as this is midwives' competence); providing food, hot, or cold drinks as needed (these evidence-based practices are allowed in most Italian hospitals, as they help the laboring woman keep her strength up); accompanying the woman in breathing; and encouraging and reassuring her. The doula can also deal with the more intimate and unpleasant aspects that can characterize labor and delivery; as Enza noted, "I remember cleaning up her vomit and she was very, very embarrassed... but I said, thank you for that...it is said that you are not a doula until you have cleaned up the vomit of a woman in labor."

Enza's words suggest how "getting your hands dirty" represents an effective initiation into the doula community. Cleaning vomit in labor means that the doula has built a deeply intimate relationship with that client. It also gives materiality to labor support, meaning that the doula is fully present at the event. Finally, through the cleansing of vomit, the doula expresses her humility and shows that she is truly at her client's service. The talent of humility has frequently emerged in the interlocutors' stories; indeed, it appears as an indispensable quality, together with patience and with the awareness of the limitations of their skills.

The interlocutors also support women whose caesarean births are scheduled, both during pregnancy and in the immediate postpartum, taking care of all the mother's needs:

> one thing we learn is to suggest to mothers who will schedule a caesarean[is] to talk to their babies and prepare them for this event ... is a way to get them into communication with the child ... On the way to

the hospital, we talk about this thing that is happening, we talk about the emotions, we invite mom and dad to tell if they are afraid, how they feel, I help the Dad to find his role in this situation. My primary goal is to help parents to feel that they are good and they are doing a great job.

(Bice)

About helping a mother who had a cesarean birth and wanted to breastfeed, Iris said:

> I went there the night of the operation … I had my bunk that I use when I do the nights, my dinner, a book… She asked me to wake her up every three hours with the breast pump ready and so I did: I woke up, I prepared it, I helped her pull up, put her legs down, I gave her the breast pump, and once I had taken the milk I went to the nursery and the midwives gave it to the baby. I also did the same on the second night. In the morning, we managed to put her in the wheelchair and went to the nursery. I will always remember the gaze of terror of other mothers, and there she suckled her child and it was very nice.

The determination of this mother, who rationally decided to manage her breastfeeding with the support of her doula, despite her need for rest and the general difficulties that a cesarean birth can cause to the body, astonished the other new mothers. Their "gaze of terror" actually includes a mix of astonishment and surprise at the courage of this mother, and of fear for her recovery, which, they believe, might be compromised by her initiative. The priority of this mother was to give breastmilk and then to breastfeed her baby, so she considered that this was the only solution to the rules of that hospital, which require new mothers to reach the nursery to breastfeed or to interact with their babies. In some Italian hospitals, rooming-in is not implemented; babies stay in the nursery all the time and mothers have to go to the nursery to spend time with the baby or to breastfeed. This organization of the obstetrics department was common in all Italian hospitals until the 1980s, whereas nowadays, rooming-in is increasingly practiced.

Finally, doula support during labor involves a *doula in seconda*, who is a backup doula available if the doula hired is suddenly unavailable. The doula in seconda is introduced to the mother by her original doula, who is responsible for creating a connection between the two women in advance of the birth, in case the backup doula is needed.

Postpartum

In the postpartum period, the doula supports the family reorganization after the arrival of the baby; she can also coordinate visits of relatives and friends, take care of tidying up the house, look after the newborn while the mother takes a moment for herself or while resting, support the client to narrate her birth story, to breastfeed, and in all her needs:

She [the mother] said, "I can do it if you help me turn around and get up" [the mother was lying in the couch] and I said, "There's no need to turn around, stay the way you are because you said you're fine in this position, let's put the baby at your height," and then I put two simple pillows, you know, two simple pillows, I raised the baby and he latched onto the breast.

(Alda)

... after giving birth…it's a world, really a world, you have to go there [the mother's house] and see, observe and then do what is needed, breastfeeding, answering questions, supporting with the first baby bath, caring of the umbilical cord, in the sense of how to do it…. Cleaning the house, preparing meals ... counseling the couple [laughs], I mean mediating between dad and mom in some circumstances ...

(Rosa)

The important thing is to be there and welcome, embrace, calm, listen, listen to and understand what they say. Not only listening but also welcoming, understanding. Because if one just listens it is not enough. Put your mom at ease and then things go well, they work out, that she's doing fine, she is good

(Lisa)

Each experience brings different needs, and doulas welcome them and adapt their activities to them. Some doulas are available to sleep at the client's home, especially during the first weeks after the delivery. In the postpartum period, the doula's role is considered by the interlocutors to be extremely important, because the hormonal changes experienced by the woman and the complexity in the redefinition of the family balance expose her to moments of extreme fragility. The doula supports the woman and the family in the case of the "baby blues," and, over time, can detect deeper symptoms and direct the new mother to competent professionals. During this period, doulas also encourage women to attend meetings with other new mothers or can organize themselves "circles of mothers," with the aim of encouraging sharing and discussion among members of a peer group and the creation of a friend support network. Finally, doulas can propose specific rituals, such as the "closing bones" massage[1] with the

---

1 This is an entire body massage that consists of wrapping the rebozo around each part of the mother's body, starting with her feet and ankles and moving up from there, and pulling the two ends of the rebozo tightly together to center the mother and help her come back to herself physically, emotionally, and spiritually. This technique works best when two people, one on each side of the mother, who is lying down, do the wrapping and then trade and pull on the ends of the shawl to literally "pull the mother together." Robbie Davis-Floyd, who had been feeling very tense and was gifted with this wrapping by two traditional midwives in Mexico, says that it "felt wonderful, like a full-body massage, and really did leave me feeling much more relaxed and centered, and not tense and scattered, as I had been before the procedure" (personal communication, June 2021).

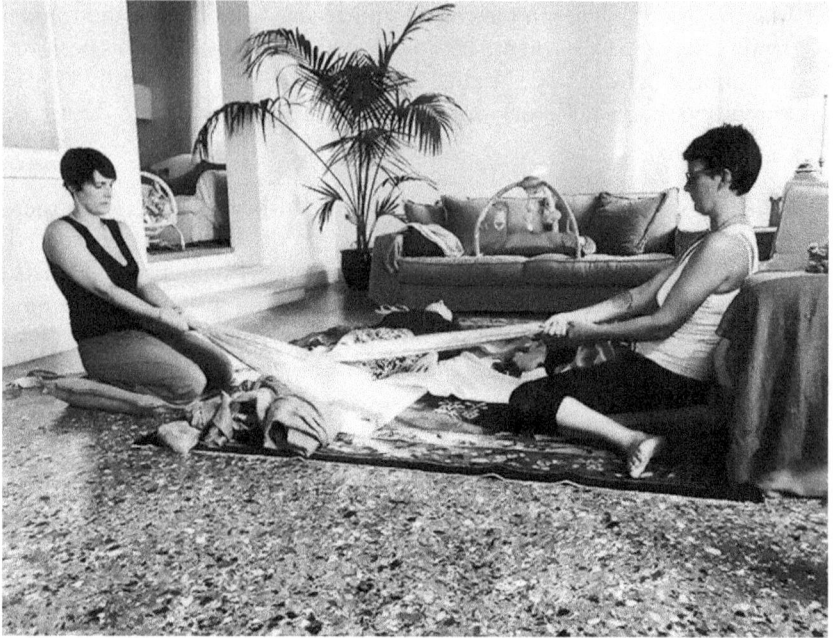

Figure 5.3 Two doulas doing a closing bones massage with a rebozo.
Source: Photograph by Davide Lipari.

rebozo (see Figure 5.3) or the farewell ceremony for the placenta, should one be held.

Types of doulas

I have described the features of doula work, but what about the *meanings* that doulas attribute to their work? The lack of institutional recognition of the doula profession reflects the difficulty of obtaining greater social recognition and spread. This indeterminacy stimulates the creation of an original professional identity. Literature has shown that in contemporary society, an individual occupies several worlds, and the professional world is only one of them (Bauman 2007; Castel 2009). However, it is on the basis of this professional world that individual life is structured as a dimension of self-realization, of subsistence, and of identification (Viteritti 2005; Gallino 2007), and this seems even more true in the case of doulas, considering the literal embodiment of their professional skills. The meanings that doulas give to their work determine the construction of the professional style that they incorporate and that they express in defining themselves. Starting from this meaning and self-definition, I have elaborated three typologies of doulas: the "progressive doula," the "philanthropic doula," and the "individualistic doula." Each type, however, has flexible boundaries and the transition from one type to another may occur as a result of events that change subjective perceptions.

The progressive doula

The progressive doula gives her practice a political–cultural meaning—as Davis-Floyd has often said, "for midwives and doulas, the professional is political" (personal communication, August 2021). This type of doula aims to activate empowerment processes in women, so they can choose and achieve the kind of pregnancy and childbirth they most want. Through the control of pregnancy and birth, the medical system oppresses women's freedom, and to redeem this situation, the progressive doulas propose an instrumental use of techno-medicine—meaning that technological interventions, such as epidurals, should only be used when women are fully informed about their benefits and risks. In all Italian hospitals, patients have to sign an "informed choice sheet" after receiving all information regarding the procedures that will be adopted. Nevertheless, the completeness of the information depends on the availability of the physician to give it, and in the more or less humanistic approach of this professional.

The progressive doula aspires to a cultural change that the transformative potential of pregnancy and childbirth can facilitate:

> … for me it has a political sense, in the sense that I believe a lot in the centrality of women during birth, and I believe that for a number of historical and social reasons, this is no longer so … I think the doula has a role to play in restoring that role to the woman … I believe that the woman can make any choice she wants as long as she is properly informed … I do not make a speech about the naturalness of childbirth, but I do make a speech about free choice, awareness, and I believe that the doula in this can do a good job both of information and of accompanying and mediation with the …hospital institution, and then I think she can make a good cultural mediation with circles, with families, with her mother-in-law in giving the right information… so that the woman can have a good experience, whether that is giving birth under a cherry tree or that is doing a scheduled caesarean birth.
>
> (Elga)

> Those who are my age … when thinking about the doula also think about the political impact in the broad sense, that is, as someone said, "birth is not a private act but a public act" … I also add political because it has implications … because the woman has to be able to choose what she wants, she wants to be anesthetized, she doesn't want to see and feel anything and see her child after 3 days, that's fine, just as it's fine

if there's a woman who wants to give birth alone, without healthcare assistance.

(Rita)

The progressive doula expands her doula training via paths that integrate her skills, preferring courses offered by institutions or associations recognized at the national level. The progressive doula considers it useful to obtain certificates supported institutionally or by public opinion, to feel her role legitimized and recognized. Obtaining these qualifications is fundamental to progressive doulas, to enable them to serve as intermediaries in institutional contexts, and to introduce themselves to clients using titles and degrees already known by the majority of the population. The progressive doula seeks to achieve majority recognition for her profession. Another characteristic of the progressive doula is a strong aptitude for founding or collaborating with associations using the doula network (personal sites or social network pages) for her self-promotion. These are doulas who have mostly embodied a professional entrepreneurial style; their maximum aspiration would be to work in the public sector. While acknowledging this as a utopian ambition, the progressive doulas say that their ideal workplace would be public hospitals, since the doula should be a professional part of the national healthcare system. Progressive doulas reference the economic savings that the healthcare system could benefit from, considering the fewer interventions and shorter labor times that the presence of a doula can facilitate. In short, they stress that doulas save the system money. It is clear to them that the presence of doulas in public hospitals, who are officially employed and on-call in those hospitals, would ensure a fixed salary for the doula and a high number of clients for her to support and empower. Progressive doulas do recognize that this way of working would preclude the development of a pre-existing relationship with the pregnant woman yet understand that deep relationships can be quickly established as the laboring woman comes rapidly to realize the benefits of the individual support the doula provides. The progressive doulas are mostly involved in the political process of achieving institutional recognition of the profile; they consider this to be a fundamental goal for the profession's legitimization. This type of doula is most common in the Italian context: around 50% of interlocutors can be defined as progressive doulas.

The philanthropic doula

The philanthropic doula considers her activity as a mission and a vocation, and the meaning she gives to it is social and supportive. Around 31% of interlocutors can be considered philanthropic doulas. These have as their primary objective, not the legitimization of the profession as the progressive doulas seek to do—though they do have a partial interest in that—but rather simply to help women and families cope gracefully with the delicate period of gestation and birth. The philanthropic doula has usually suffered a traumatic experience during the perinatal period, and this experience pushes her to do her utmost to ensure that the loneliness and the bewilderment that she has experienced do not have to happen to other women. Supporting other childbearers allows the philanthropic doula to ease, albeit symbolically, her own suffering, to conceptually rewrite her own birth story. These philanthropic doulas feel empowered to take care of their clients, developing, on occasion, a female network of help and support in order to fill any social, institutional, or family gap. The philanthropic doula speaks of love, help, and support and calls for an ideal of sisterhood to which women should aspire, indicating with this term a willingness to collaborate and to provide mutual help. In lieu of professional recognition, personal recognition by her clients confers the type of legitimacy to which the philanthropic doula aspires:

> ... it's like a vocation, I feel it as a vocation, as a way to make the mother and the child feel good, and then improve the family a little.
>
> (Susi)

> The doula helps ... to help, I don't find any other meaning, I see it just as help.
>
> (Alda)

> ... personally I don't feel like it is a profession, more like a vocation ... I realized what it means for a mother to give birth in a big hospital [where there are many new mothers and health care professionals don't have time to provide care in a welcoming way] because I saw how a mother can be left alone in that situation ... the doula perhaps exists because there is a void.
>
> (Nina)

To expand her training, the philanthropic doula chooses diversified paths, without caring much about who the trainers are nor about the educational institution. She is simply moved by the desire to learn useful tools to help mothers; for example, she attends courses on breastfeeding or on babywearing and/or learns techniques such as the harmonization/psychological integration of scars (see Chapter 4). The philanthropic doula occasionally uses the Internet to promote herself, prefers working in her residential area, organizing meetings and conferences, and creating collaborations with associations and with shops that sell maternity items. She also collaborates with institutions; an example is the free-of-charge collaboration among four doulas and a prison in Rome, in which the doulas support the pregnant prisoners during labor and birth. Additionally, the philanthropic doula participates in conferences and seminars offered by other organizations with the aim of expanding her regional network. This type of doula appears to be only partially interested in working in the public sector: as for the progressive doula, the aspects that attract her interest in public hospital work include the possibility of helping a large number of women and benefiting from a fixed salary. The less attractive aspect for the philanthropic doula is the risk of the establishment of a rigid definition of the doula, which the institutionalization of the doula would require, and the consequent limitation of the doula's autonomy. The strategies and strong relationships that the philanthropic doula has developed in her region allow her to practice even without national recognition and legitimization.

The individualistic doula

This category includes doulas who have given to their practices an individual and personal meaning. Despite the differences among them, what unites the individualistic doulas is an eclectic attitude and a particular charisma, which elevates them to the position of "the model to be followed." This is the smallest group among the interlocutors, accounting for around 19%. These individualistic doulas have a high level of previous education; they are the founders of schools or those who create other training courses, or they are doulas who are recognized within associations for their charismatic personalities. They often define themselves not only as doulas but also as "guardians of birth," "mothers' assistants," "birthkeepers," etc. They are doulas who also deal with parental education and meditation, and who generally consider doula work not as a profession nor as a vocation, but as a lifestyle:

> For me to do this thing, to go to someone's house, listen to them carefully and welcome what they tell you... to not trigger the mechanism of judgment, but say "I'm here for you" has become educational of how I treat myself ... really it has become something that is much more ... while before I felt like a social activist, now it seems to me that the strongest thing I'm doing is changing *me*.
>
> (Mina)

> It's my life, it's my life, because it coincides with my life, I don't have a private and a professional life, it's absolutely my life and I do it also inevitably, I can't do it in every moment of my life.
>
> (Elsa)

> There is this thing here that is very strong in motherhood... this sense of inheritance, legacy, this need of tradition, of tradition as to pass on as inheritance, but also as to contradict ... and the doula is just this, both the ability to inhabit the maternal way of being, but also to contradict it if we want. The doula offers you both because she is the third subject

between mother and daughter...that is the position from which you look at the mother-daughter relationship, both your relationship within yourself, and the relationship of the people you follow, you accompany ... I think of doulas as an archetype, and the archetype is to be the mother of herself ... in fact I think that a doula can constellate in a woman and with a woman this ability, mothering the mother allows her to feel able to be a mother and then mothering herself ... this as an archetype in my opinion has never been studied—I would like to do that sooner or later.

(Mina)

Each individualistic doula follows her own training and in-depth trajectory, ranging from seminars and workshops of a scientific or medical nature to meditation paths that stem from Oriental philosophies. The issue of individual responsibility comes up very frequently in the narratives told by these individualistic doulas: it is a question of responsibility toward oneself, to realize one's own potential, to satisfy one's own well-being, and to promote the same process in the mothers they care for. The individualistic doula uses the Internet sporadically and only to promote her training courses or the seminars she organizes. These occasions are her main promotional strategies, as they give her the opportunity to express her charismatic personality and consequently to attract more clients.

In contrast to the progressive and the philanthropic doula, the public sector as a possible professional space does not interest the individualistic doula, since she thinks that mothers need to have the possibility of choosing their own professional care providers, and the formal introduction of the doula into an institution like the hospital would compromise her ability to practice as she wishes. Furthermore, the rigid definition of the profile and the restrictions on her practice that the hospital would require are seen by individualistic doulas as major restrictions on their professional autonomy, just as they are by the philanthropic doulas. For the same reasons, the individualistic doulas consider an institutional recognition of their profession both unnecessary and dangerous for their freedom of practice. The doulas of this group benefit from a strong acknowledgment of their efficacy both among mothers and among other doulas; they base their legitimacy on this recognition.

Intra-professional relations

In the previous sections, I have shown how the different meanings that doulas attribute to their work determine the construction of three different professional styles: progressive, philanthropic, and individualistic. This heterogeneity is one of the major reasons why Italian doulas cannot unite and speak with one unified voice:

... at the moment there are different, contrasting visions, the range of shades is quite wide, even the different models of schools that have arisen ... at this time one of the obstacles is also the difficulty of creating a constructive dialogue, as the various associations and schools of doulas in many cases fail to dialogue or do so with great difficulty.

(Clio)

In the last meeting we had between trainers [of different doula schools], we asked ourselves who the doula is and we didn't even agree that it was a woman. For me there is no doubt. For me the doula can only be a woman, not a man.

(Irma)

I had to realize this ... It's so nice to say in words, "we're sisters, we work together," then in fact these are all big lies, each one wants to emerge, each one wants to be the queen and this job is not a job where there's a queen. If we want to recognize that there is a person who has more leadership, more charisma, and more experience, ok, but she must not stand on a pedestal, no, absolutely not.

(Edda)

Abbott (1988) states that internal differentiation in a professional group can have profound consequences in the system of professions. The effects vary according to the internal structure involved. In particular, Abbott identifies four possibilities: (1) the internal differences are incorporated into the intra-professional status, (2) they are incorporated by dividing the clients, (3) they are incorporated by a division of labor, or (4) they are incorporated according to the careers of the professionals. These different structures are not separate; indeed, they reinforce each other. From the accounts of doulas emerges a work organization that gives to the presidents of associations, and in general to the executive boards, the power to make fundamental decisions concerning the definition, the training, and the path for obtaining an institutional recognition of the doula profile. The association leaders generally comprise their founders, their trainers, and their most experienced doulas. It is in the narratives of the doulas who hold executive roles that the elements of divergence of the professional group emerge most strongly. However, these elements do not seem to have particularly affected the development of the profession.

Internal differentiation within a professional group can create disturbances to the system of professions or be absorbed by it (Abbott 1988). In my view, analysis of the current experience of doulas, and by extension of any emerging professional group, requires an advancement in theorization. The internal differences among the different types of doulas were not absorbed by the professional doula system and did not generate particular disturbances in that system. The only other professional group involved is the professional group of midwives, as I will explore in Chapter 6. In general, I can affirm that the system of professions surrounding the doula profession simply did not have the possibility of being disturbed by the differences among doulas, since Italian doulas as a whole have consciously adopted a compensation strategy that allows them to interact with each other and with the other professional groups in a cohesive way, despite their differing perspectives:

> Each doula behaves as she wishes but having the awareness that there is a shared feminine knowledge, that there is sisterhood, this is important.
> (Dina)

> For me the importance of the network between doulas … I believe that our first task is "to sister," to learn to be among women and to be there with a certain quality, which is that of acceptance, welcome, listening, and mutual respect in diversity.
> (Mina)

> The other thing that made me very passionate is the contact with other women, to be part of a very large group, not simply a group of people who meet physically, but a group I would say also extended to the whole Italian territory, women for women, and this re-emergence, that immersion for me in the female dimension has fueled my passion.
> (Mara)

> Then I happened to be interviewed by newspapers and magazines—just this morning I got contacted by one of them for an interview—[and in these interviews] I have always mentioned all the associations, and this is for me is sisterhood and it is important in fact to demonstrate it.
> (Edda)

Thus, we can see that the internal differentiation is obviated by doulas through an embodied rhetoric. *Sisterhood* and belonging to the same group constitute strong elements of cohesion. In their activities, doulas recognize the importance of being supportive of women in general, and of each other, no matter who belongs to what association. This group solidarity is nourished by the frequent exchanges that take place during seminars or training workshops, or within private groups in the social networks. If a doula asks for suggestions and support in reference to her practice on one of the social networking groups, she always receives a great deal of feedback from other doulas, regardless of the association to which they belong. Online interactions also involve those who hold leadership roles in associations. *Chi la doula la vince* is a joking play on words, on the Italian expression *Chi la dura la vince,* which is translated into English as "Who tries and tries again finally succeeds." That joke and the expression "Keep calm, I'm a doula" are slogans created by doulas to encourage each other, define a working style, and act as strong cohesive elements for this professional group. Solidarity takes shape also through the creation of special gifts: see Figure 5.4.

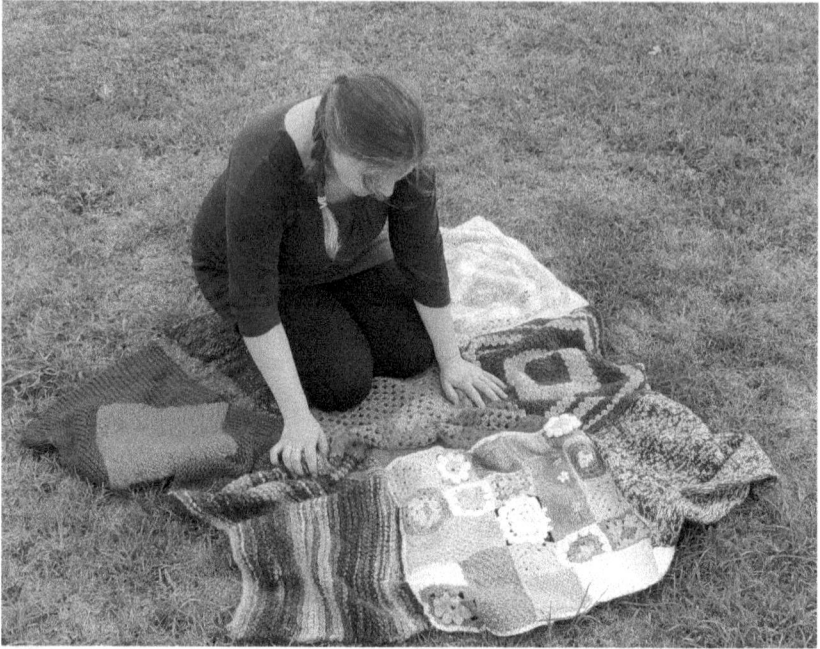

Figure 5.4 A doula with her special blanket. During a doula training of the
Association Mondo Doula, a doula shared with her classmate that she
often felt cold and lonely. Other participants decided to create a blanket
for her. Each one knitted a piece of blanket; even those who couldn't knit
asked for support from friends and relatives who could. Once finished,
all the pieces were knitted together to give physical and symbolic warmth
to the doula.

Source: Photograph by Marco Coltro.

Therefore, I consider that internal differentiation within a group can
cause disruption to the system of professions, can absorb disruption of the
system, or cannot affect the system at all. The prerequisite for the system
not to be affected is the ability of the group to adopt a strategy that gives
a lower value to the elements that diverge and a higher value on those that
generate cohesion. Diminishing the importance of differences and adopting a
rhetoric that, by appealing to shared values and to meetings and exchanges,
avoids internal crises are the characteristics of this third possible outcome of
internal differentiation.

Conclusion

The doula profession aims to respond to the need for support of new
and becoming mothers. The establishment of a specific work niche—a

jurisdiction—has been carried out in two ways: on the one hand, the doula combines in a single person "bits and pieces" of tasks and roles that have been traditionally covered by family members or different professional figures such as babysitters and live-in nannies or au pairs (for those who can afford them). On the other hand, the doula satisfies childbearers' needs in an innovative way: normally, the person seeking professional help goes to that professional's office, yet the doula as a professional goes to the home and offers listening, care, empowerment, and in general pays special attention to the emotional dimensions of women and families who are living the perinatal experience. Although doulas attribute different meanings to their work and hold differing values and perspectives, these elements do not seem to be limiting the development of the profession. The adoption of a rhetoric of sisterhood and solidarity that embodies these fundamental aspects of the doula profession can be interpreted as a strategy to overcome differences and strengthen bonds that can ensure the ongoing development of the professional doula in Italy.

6   Doulas and midwives

In his analysis of the system of professions, Abbott (1988) states that one of the fundamental aspects in a profession's history is inscribed in the relationships that one profession entertains with the others, and in the disputes surrounding the conquest of the relative jurisdiction. The claim to full jurisdiction is only one of the possible settlements of a jurisdictional conflict. In general, this is the goal of all other types of settlements, since every profession aims for a body of work over which it has complete control. Following Abbott, professions may have to accept a variety of alternative settlements to develop themselves and solve possible conflicts:

1   **Subordination.** One profession becomes dominant, subordinating the others. This is, for example, what happened between architects and draftsmen; the latter are essential part of the architectural practice, but their work derives from the former.

2   **Division of labor.** The professions divide one jurisdiction into two interdependent parts, and occasionally they can share an area without a division of labor. In this sense, architects have full jurisdiction over the design of buildings, but they divide their work with engineers, whereas 100 years ago, architects were responsible for everything, including engineering.

3   **Intellectual.** A profession retains control of the cognitive knowledge of an area but allows practice by competitors. This has been the situation of psychiatry and psychology since World War II. For decades, psychiatry maintained its preeminence through allowing only MDs to lay claim to the field of mental health. Yet because psychiatrists were expensive and relied primarily on Freudian analysis for a very long time, there was an open space for non-MD psychologists and social workers to fill using other techniques, showing that the "owners" of a particular jurisdiction can lose a large part of their professional "territory"—in this case, mental health—to another, overlapping profession. This is precisely what midwives fear about doulas.

4   **Advisory jurisdiction.** One profession seeks a legitimate right to interpret or partially modify actions that another takes within its own

DOI: 10.4324/9781003165934-7

jurisdiction. Medicine, for example, has expanded its jurisdiction into child behavior in this way. Doctors transformed advice into diseases and treated children with drugs—just as psychiatrists have transformed mental illnesses into pathologies and treated them with drugs, which psychologists do not.

5 **Workplace settlement.** Professions divide the jurisdiction not through a division of labor, but through a division in the type of clients served. For example, in 19th-century England, physicians treated the upper classes, and "barber-surgeons" and midwives treated the middle and lower classes.

To Abbott's list above, Adams (2007) adds "cooperation" as a possible outcome between professional groups that share similarity in size, outlook, and legislative status, and whose areas of expertise overlap. This is the case in the Netherlands (Cheyney et al. 2019) and New Zealand (Georges and Daellenbach 2019), where midwives and obstetricians cooperate instead of competing. Midwives represent the professional group with which doulas interact most, which, as highlighted in Chapter 2, has developed strategies to prevent the emergence and practice of doulas. However, this scene is characterized by considerable complexity—by cooperation as well as conflict. Thus, this chapter aims to analyze how doulas are defining their presence within the system of maternity care professions, most especially in relation to midwives.

Italian midwives in context

The history of the midwifery profession in Italy is marked by remarkable discontinuities that alternate periods of relative autonomy with periods of domination and subordination (Spina 2014). The figure of the midwife is undoubtedly among the oldest in history. Ancient Greece and Rome recognized famous midwives and held in high regard the exercise of midwifery, which was separate from the medical profession. For centuries, medicine paid only theoretical attention to midwifery, delegating the practice to women, mostly uneducated (Pancino 1984). In the 16th century, a new interest in medicine and anatomical studies spread in Italy and Europe and began to prefigure the possibility that men could attend births. It was only around the middle of the 18th century that birth assistance, until then considered a matter of women, linked to nature, fate, and magical–ritual knowledge, became an object of medical interest. The medical specializations of obstetrics and gynecology were born. Men began to deal with pregnancy and childbirth, resulting in a transformation in the cultural ways of conceiving those events, and changing the basis of the legitimacy of the practitioners appointed to assist women (Filippini 1995). The midwife was relegated to the assistance of physiological delivery and trained to recognize the symptoms of pathology in order to request a doctor's intervention. This triggered the socio-professional decline of the midwife, who started to increasingly take a subordinate role compared to the doctor (Spina 2009). During the 18th century, high infant and childbirth mortality captured the attention of European governments, which addressed the problem by investing in training: schools for midwives were born. In Italy, between 1757 and 1779, 13 midwifery schools were created; the first was in Turin (1732), followed by Bologna (1757), Milan (1767), Venice (1770), etc. (Filippini 2017).

However, the institutionalization of training courses did not eliminate the presence of the traditional Italian midwife, called *levatrice*, who had been assisting births in Italy for centuries, thanks to her experiential training via apprenticeships with more experienced midwives. For a time, the levatrice coexisted with the newer, more modern, professionally and didactically trained midwives. The coexistence of professionally trained midwives and levatrici continued until the beginning of the 20th century, when there occurred a stiffening in the access to the professional group through the introduction of tests and examinations by the state. The age limit for accessing institutional educational paths was decreased to allow younger women to become midwives, and the duration of the training was extended to prevent the remaining older levatrici from institutionalizing their position.

The 19th century was a century of controversy for Italian midwives: on the one hand, there was a proliferation of institutions responsible for midwives' training; on the other, the levatrici were continuously readmitted within the official circuit through state decrees, dictated by the need for birth attendants (Pancino 1984). This situation fostered the rancor of the "educated" midwives, who, united in federations and supported by a part of the medical professional group, rose against the levatrici. To acquire support and legitimacy, the institutionalized midwives of the late 19th century chose to support physicians and the medicalization of birth, moving away from a popular tradition hostile to this process that had characterized the levatrici approach. This choice failed to achieve the desired advantages of a substantial recognition of professional midwifery; on the contrary, it dragged midwives into a hierarchical system, limiting their autonomy and obliging them to perform functions subsidiary to the medical profession (Spina 2009). Today, I wonder what would have happened if the professional midwives and the levatrici had joined forces to establish midwifery as an autonomous profession with official and substantial sociocultural recognition. Such an alliance did occur in Canada in the early 1980s, at a time when midwifery did not exist as a recognized profession in Canada. To create that profession, the "lay" homebirth midwives of Ontario—mostly, like the levatrici, trained by apprenticeship—joined forces with the Ontario nurse–midwives, who had been trained as such in other countries but were unable to practice as midwives in Canada, only as nurses. Their alliance culminated in the 1993 formal legalization of "direct-entry" midwifery (midwives who are directly trained in midwifery and do not go through nursing education first) in Ontario as an autonomous profession; today direct-entry midwives (called RMs—registered midwives), usually trained in four-year university programs, are legal across Canada (see Bourgealt et al. 2004). Had such an alliance been established in Italy between the levatrici and the professional midwives, the Italian midwifery profession might be stronger and might benefit from knowledge derived from actual experience and not only from biomedical science.

In the 20th century, with the advent of the fascist regime in Italy, midwives obtained institutional recognition through the creation of a "professional order" in 1927. To exercise the profession, midwives needed to attend a specific training and pass a state exam, after which they could be registered in the "professional order," which is a statal public body that assures the competence and professionalism of its members. Although in 1934, a law on health defined the figure of the midwife as auxiliary and supportive to the main figures (doctor–surgeon, pharmacist, veterinarian), between 1910 and 1940, the midwife's public function evolved, thanks to the social legitimation obtained through the institution of the *condotta ostetrica*. The midwives condotte were community midwives appointed by the state who ensured maternity care for all women, especially for those who lived in the countryside or on mountains or islands far from hospitals. Usually, the condotta worked alone; her support was requested by husbands or other relatives when the mother-to-be started labor. The condotta went to the woman's home and stayed with her until the baby was born ("*Nati in casa*"—*Born at home*, by Giuliana Musso and Massimo Somaglino, is a fascinating theater performance in which the stories of three condotta midwives are described, together with their difficulties in reaching birthing women through rain, wind, and snow, and supporting them, sometimes for days). Only in emergency cases did the condotta ask for medical support; in those cases, the husbands or other relatives had to reach the home of the closest doctor to deliver the midwife's request for assistance.

The post-war years, characterized by an economic boom and urbanization, marked the final entry of childbirth into the hospital. The hospitalization of births involved the massive entrance of the condotta midwife into the hospital and brought about the decline of this kind of midwife, until her final disappearance through the health reform that established the National Health System. The autonomy that had characterized the condotta midwife midwife gave way to subordination (Spina 2009). In 1976, the midwifery profession was opened to men, and in 1980, the Fnopo (National Federation of Midwives) asked to transform midwifery schools into degree-granting universities. Through the reform of the teaching system (Law 341/90), midwives' educational programs were transformed into academic courses. At this stage, the hospitalization of births and the increasing medicalization process can be considered co-responsible for the socio-professional decline of midwifery and the strengthening of gynecology/obstetrics as a medical discipline and profession.

The 1990s saw a long series of law reforms that affected midwives: the professional profile with its areas of competence and responsibility was defined; and the training path to become a midwife was reorganized through the establishment of a three-year university degree course. Despite the statal official recognition, midwives continue to experience medical dominance and subordination (Spina 2014) in the hospital, since no tools are available to monitor the respect of professional tasks and boundaries between the two professional groups. In other words, midwives do have official recognition, they are autonomous by law, but in the hospital, doctors supervise midwives' work, and they have to ask for the doctor's approval for much of what they do. This supervision is discretionary, because it depends on each doctor; there are doctors that leave more freedom to midwives, while others want to supervise their every action.

Hence, the midwifery profession in Italy is characterized by strong ambiguities: the statal recognition coexists with a lack of real autonomy for professional midwives and a lack of recognition by the population. When Italian women get pregnant, they commonly choose a gynecologist/ obstetrician as their primary healthcare provider, even in cases of normal physiological pregnancy, despite the fact that according to the law, the competent professional in this arena is the midwife, and gynecologists/ obstetricians should take care only of pathological pregnancies and births.

Rather than growing their profession on their own, as the doulas are doing, Italian midwives, like most of those in other European countries, have had little say in their professionalization process, which instead has been imposed from above (McClelland 1990) and implemented through external legislative interventions rather than via strategies put in place by the midwives themselves (Spina 2014), as the Canadian midwives did and as Italian doulas are seeking to do. This long path has been characterized by a lack of internal cohesion, especially in reference to the deep dualism that contrasts hospital and "freelance" midwives, who attend births in homes and freestanding birth centers.

Nowadays in Italy, there are around 17,000 midwives, who can work as freelance (about 3% of the professional group) or are employed in the National Health System, in hospitals or in public community centers. These centers are called in Italian *consultorio familiare*; they are public centers that offer healthcare and social support to families, especially dealing with motherhood and parenthood. Midwives, gynecologists, social workers, psychologists, and nurses work in these public community centers. In addition, some midwives are involved in teaching as professors in the midwifery university degree programs, and as health and sex educators.

Community midwives who work in consultori familiari can serve as the primary caregivers throughout the perinatal process of physiological pregnancies or can support obstetricians in case of pathological pregnancies.

Moreover, they organize trainings for pregnant women and perform simple diagnostic exams, such as the Pap test, and support new mothers during breastfeeding.

Midwives who work in hospitals can carry out maternity ward activities or can work in the delivery room; this division of labor depends on the organizational autonomy of each hospital structure. When carrying out delivery room activities, they have various tasks, from the monitoring of the labor to the delivery. When the birth is physiological, it is supposed to be entirely managed by midwives, who, again, are officially the professionals responsible for this process. Nevertheless, this law provision is disregarded in most cases, since almost all hospitals require that at the time of delivery, the obstetrician must be present. This requirement further limits the autonomy of midwives, who are thereby dispossessed of their delivery skills. The level of substantial autonomy of midwives in the hospital depends on several factors, such as past experience, personal values and beliefs related to the birth process, original and acquired social capital, and the personalities of both midwives and doctors (Spina 2009).

"Freelance" midwives are usually the primary caregivers throughout the perinatal process, from pregnancy to postpartum. Many freelance midwives have previously worked in hospitals, where they have acquired experience but decided to leave because they did not share the hospital's rigidly medicalized approach. They usually organize trainings and meetings for mothers-to-be, in order to help them envision pregnancy and birth in a holistic way. In their activities, freelance midwives respect statal guidelines, which, for example, foresaw the presence of two midwives during home births. They can also work in freestanding birth centers that are managed entirely by them. Freelance midwives are private professionals; their work is not covered by statal funding; and this is one of the reasons why many women cannot benefit from their support. However, some regions reimburse partially or totally the home births of those women who choose a freelance midwife as their primary healthcare provider.

Midwives' representations of doulas

Midwives' narratives about doulas reflect the duality of positions within the professional group of midwives, as characterized in the analysis of Spina (2009). In the following sections, I will deepen the two poles that characterize the midwife interlocutors' representations of doulas.

Doulas as liars and charlatans

In the accounts of midwives, mainly those of hospital and institutional representatives of the professional group, we find similar attitudes toward doulas. A first dimension mentioned by midwives refers to doula trainings:

What kind of schools do doulas attend? What do they [learn]? ... We talk about professionalization, but what school do they have? What body of knowledge do they have? They go to schools created by individual deficient midwives that allow them to exist, because if they wouldn't train doulas, they won't exist.

(Noemi)

... in my opinion, in order to be considered professionals, they should have a somewhat more important training, even in terms of time, a little longer.

(Linda)

In these quotations from midwives, we can see that the training of doulas is misconceived by midwives to be without a specific body of knowledge, too short, and lacking strong statal recognition and regulation similar to those of midwives; these lacks seem to midwives to make it impossible for the doula to define herself as a professional. The split between groups of midwives is evident in the first quotation above. Midwives who train doulas are considered "deficient" by their midwifery colleagues. This rift represents not just a duality of opinions or operational methodologies but also threatens the midwives' group. Therefore, the scenario appears complex: within the midwifery profession, there are professionals who, by providing tools and knowledge to doulas, appear to compromise the midwives' professional group. This threat, mainly felt by institutional representatives, seemed to call for a strong stance (see Chapter 2), to the extent that the suspension of a midwife who taught in a doula training program was considered exemplary by other midwives. Bruna, a midwife, in accusing that midwife of teaching in that doula training program for the money, said, "Behind it there is an economic return and that is clearly the reason why people put themselves in certain situations ... It's not good for a colleague to sell pearls to swine." Bruna's expression about selling "pearls to swine" clearly illustrates her negative conceptions of doulas—conceptions also shared by many other Italian midwives.

Professional groups defend themselves not only by coercively managing internal threats but also by acting simultaneously to delegitimize external threats:

the doula is part of the midwife ... that is, the midwife is automatically a doula, only that the midwife can act even better ... I think that doulas are frustrated failed midwives. I see them as if I could not pass the midwife test to enter the university course and then I invent to do the doula ... understood?

(Gioia)

... some colleagues tell me that doulas support mothers in interpreting blood test results ... they gave me their names.

(Adele)

... why do we perceive them [doulas] so badly? After all, because they are part of a world that is not real, it is not the delivery room, it is not the hospital, where you work in a certain way.

(Bruna)

There is no need for charlatan people, nor need for chatty people, nor even for people who find work like this, at this time when there is a tremendous fight [for money] because there is no work ... They are smart ... have changed their sites for a month now, have changed a lot because they are looking for any form of communication that can't give rise to think that they perform a health profession ... They have their lobby, they're backed by a lobby for sure, by a strong group, even politically, because if you think that they managed to have the space on the news, on Tg1 [the major channel of national public television] ... When you do interviews with them, they tell you that they don't attend births: they tell us lies! Because I have names and surnames of doulas who assist alone in labor, who assist women at home, understood?! So, they are also liars ... then they are recommended well, but surely the forefathers of this thing here are people of the bourgeoisie who have ways to acquire a whole series of things, they are scum, understand?! ... with these radical chic philosophies they get hold of.

(Noemi)

In the representations of these midwives, the delegitimization of doulas serves to create an enemy to fight; it is well known that sharing a common enemy facilitates group cohesion. According to the midwives, the profile of the doula emerged as a consequence of the economic and social crisis that had struck Italy in the previous years, but the doula is actually without skills, envious of the midwives—a midwife "wannabe"—and willing to lie and cheat to succeed. Although most of the interlocutors have never had the opportunity to discuss or collaborate with doulas, the gossip in hospital corridors or the stories told by colleagues are sufficient to discredit the figure to those who have never even met her. Midwives' discourses follow those put in place in the social construction of the "Other" as an enemy. Like migrants, who are ontologically considered to be enemies because they are seen as threats to the very foundation of the state system (Dal Lago 2004), the doula is seen as a challenge to the very existence of the midwifery profession. As Paolo Friere showed long ago in the *Pedagogy of the* Oppressed (1970), oppressed groups tend to fight the groups underneath them rather than those above them in the societal hierarchy because those "underdogs" (the doulas) are reachable, while the "top dogs" (the obstetricians) are not. Just so did certified nurse–midwives (CNMS) in the U.S.A., who are primarily hospital-based and subordinated to obstetricians, fight certified professional midwives (CPMs), who only attend births in homes and freestanding birth centers, for decades—until they finally came to understand Friere's logic, stopped coding each other as the "Other" and the "enemy," and began to work together, as they do now, to the great benefit of both groups (see Davis-Floyd and Johnson 2006 and the website "www.usmera.org"). The transformation of doulas into enemies is the means used by some midwives to symbolically delegitimize the doulas' perceived desire to take over the midwives' territory. The strategies used to pursue this aim explicitly include the adoption of derogatory terminology, as shown in Noemi's quote above. The prejudices, rumors, and urban legends that midwives circulate about doulas constitute the symbolic resources through which they strengthen their professional group, as does the creation of an ontological enemy:

> Mine is a profession of help, it is based on the relationship of help and the fact that comes out this doula, who strips off the dress of the health professional and puts on the dress of the relationship professional pisses me off even more—excuse the curse word. Why do they want to deplete my job, you know? ... This fragmentation or this division of labor into empathic part and technical part has no sense and is unacceptable. A genuine, serious midwife who has studied and understood the scientific value of the profession cannot accept the doula, cannot accept them, because this means being deprived of her role. Then it no longer makes sense that the midwife exists.
>
> (Noemi)

> ... gynecologists enter our field a lot ... unfortunately we are really attacked on all fronts, because we have gynecologists who deal with physiology and it makes no sense that they deal with physiology, but they do ... they take that slice from us [midwives], and now doulas are gonna start getting another slice ... and what's left for us? We have nothing left.
>
> (Linda)

Thus, midwives appear unwilling to share part of their jurisdiction with doulas, fearing the extinction of their profession. If doulas will become the competent professionals of emotional support, and doctors will take care of both physiological and pathological pregnancies and births, midwives believe that they would be destined to disappear. This fear and the awareness of a controversial history prompt midwives to build walls—professional "silos"—to defend their boundaries. The considerable differences between the two professional groups—midwives and doulas—in terms of size, regulation, and social legitimacy are not considered by midwives, nor is the fact that doulas hold midwives in high regard. What matters to many Italian midwives is to stop the advance of "the enemy," since the symbolic capital of the midwives is related to the cultural, social, and economic capital of doulas—which appears to midwives to threaten their own symbolic capital (Schinkel and Noordegraaf 2011).

Midwives as important supports for mothers

The narratives of other midwives, mainly freelance and community midwives, differ from those of professional and institutional representatives and hospital colleagues. Here, I present some of these differing perspectives from such midwives:

> ... It is important to give value to doulas, because if they are developing it means that there's a need and I believe that they can support us [midwives] in the continuity of assistance and the support of the physiology of motherhood ... I believe that the doula can be a great support for women, even during labor if necessary ... in my opinion she is very related to the postpartum, to tell you the truth.
>
> (Giada)

> With the doula I worked twice, once in the postpartum ... A new mother asked me about a nanny, I introduced her to a doula, and I told her the difference. While in the other case I was hired from a mother-to-be who wanted to labor mainly at home and then deliver in the hospital, actually in that case I was called by the doula and I went with her to this mother's house and then we accompanied her to the hospital—the relationship went very well.
>
> (Lucia)

> ... during the time I was working in Emilia Romagna [an Italian region where this midwife interlocutor had met doulas] for me it was a good thing, so much that when I saw that here, in my area, there was the training to become doula, I thought of attending it ... but then I didn't do it for lack of money and time.
>
> (Carla)

As these quotations illustrate, doulas are recognized and valued by some midwives, especially those who have had personal experience with them. This willingness and openness to collaborate with and promote the doula on the parts of some midwives marks a clear division within the midwives' professional group and opens new configurations of the two professional fields:

> ... someone says it's a thing for Americans because they don't have midwives like we do ... It's true that healthcare welfare systems are different, but Western social models are similar ... I'd like doulas to be institutionalized. What I don't like is that it's only for people who can afford it, but I don't think *anyone* likes that.
>
> (Agata)

In addition to socially and symbolically recognizing the value of the doula, Agata's words show her desire—shared by other midwives—for a substantial institutional recognition for doulas. These freelance midwives do not see doulas as their enemies but rather as possible allies in pursuing the ultimate goal of the midwife's work: to ensure a good experience of pregnancy, childbirth, and motherhood to all women. However, these midwives specify that "cooperation" needs to be clearly defined:

> … we are two different professions, surely there are overlapping points, while others are not overlapping at all.
>
> (Lucia)

> … it depends on what role the doula should play … [that role] should certainly not clash with the role of the midwife. If the roles are distinct and intersect with each other, who will benefit from it is the mother. If, on the other hand, you start arguing about skills, you don't go anywhere and the friction comes out and whoever loses is the mother. It's supposed to be a team job.
>
> (Carla)

> … there is room for everyone, but we have to define boundaries and roles. Boundaries and roles must be respected. They must be respected for the good especially of the mother.
>
> (Adele)

Curi (2012) points out how the term "border," in one of its meanings, evokes a contact, a meeting: in the act of separating two entities, the border can also bring them together. And it is precisely this encounter, this contact with the "other," that allows "us" to define and recognize ourselves. It is not simply a question of defining a role. It goes further: the daily actions situated in the working practices actually strengthen the belonging that characterizes the identity. The construction of the identity, in fact, seems to be based on the identification and definition of an "otherness" (Toffanin 2015). In recognizing and defining the work of doulas, midwives prove their awareness of belonging to another professional community. It's as if this group of midwives would affirm:

> I am a midwife and you are a doula, and we cooperate with each other because we recognize that we do different things that are sometimes interconnected. We can help each other to help the laboring woman, because her wellbeing and that of her baby are the goals we both seek to accomplish.

Therefore, this group of midwives appears willing to move in a different direction than the institutional representatives and their hospital colleagues, operationalizing a division of work that in fact could divide the jurisdiction between the two professions in helpful ways:

> ... many midwives are afraid to see a slice of their work taken away ... there are colleagues jealous of their work ... the speeches I heard are "these doulas here take away our work" ... in my opinion it is not so ... the birth is not mine; the birth event is not mine ... And if there is a figure that can support the woman and even just walk into a house and say "You are good, you're doing very well," without judging ... she is welcome! And above all ... to be able to go home to support those women that I can't see because they don't come to the community center.
>
> (Ester)

> The whole battle against doulas has always seemed weird to me.
>
> (Agata)

> There is a national midwives' federation, but I do not participate in its activities, I am part of it because I must be there to be allowed to work, but I do not "feel" it.
>
> (Adele)

> It is not the approach I would like my federation to have towards these supportive figures.
>
> (Giada)

Spina (2009) has highlighted the lack of internal cohesion within the professional group of midwives, the partial sense of belonging that Adele expresses, and the lack of participation in the activities of the national federation. According to Spina, representative bodies are seen as strong and closed silos, self-referential, and unwilling to seek the approval of their members that could legitimize their activities. The stress that the figure of the doula brings to the midwifery profession seems to further confirm the deep rift within this professional group. The absence of shared goals prevents the development of a sense of common belonging that might enable Italian midwives to advance their profession (Sarfatti Larson 1977). Moreover, the internal fragmentation gives space for expansion and affirmation to doulas, who are cohesive in desiring recognition and legitimacy.

I argue that instead of fighting doulas, Italian midwives should fight against their subordination to obstetricians and for real implementation of the laws that (at least on paper) have put them in charge of normal physiological births; in these ways, they could reclaim their autonomy in birth attendance. Certain obstetricians, not doulas, are midwives' real enemies—the ones who deprive them of the autonomy that they are officially supposed to have. Yet as Friere showed, it is always easier to fight the group below you in the hierarchy rather than the one above. Should Italian midwives become autonomous and in full charge of the births they attend, their value as maternity care providers would become unquestioned, and they would not need to fear a doula takeover of their functions.

Doulas' representations of midwives

The doulas' representations of midwives appear uniformly positive. Their narratives highlight a respect for professional boundaries, recognition, and enhancement of midwives, as illustrated in these quotations from doulas:

> … It is very clear that the role of the midwife is one thing, the role of the doula is another, they can cooperate together because we say that the woman must be at the center, must be helped … to do the good for the mother there can be several professionals.
>
> (Vera)

> … We strongly suggest women to contact the midwife, that is, when they say "ah but I have a gynecologist", we all say "but you know that if your pregnancy is physiological you can be supported by a midwife instead of the gynecologist?" A lot of women don't know that, and that's a big problem for midwives.
>
> (Rita)

> I hold the midwife's work in high regard … their professional history has been very mistreated, because they have suffered what women often suffer professionally.
>
> (Leda)

> … the situation of midwives is the factor that is urgent to change … The guidelines of our Ministry of Health must be applied, because they state that the midwife is the central figure in the health care of women … it should be midwives to assess when a pregnancy is straying from physiology and then they should call, consult, or send the woman to other professionals who are more suitable to each woman.
>
> (Elsa)

> …women often don't know who to ask … I am often asked for information that should be the midwife's responsibility, but the use of a midwife as a figure in charge of maternity, birth and physiology of pregnancy is not taken for granted and in the collective imagination, the midwife is not the competent figure … it is the gynecologist, but in truth it is not so."
>
> (Gaia)

Doulas' accounts recognize the lack of midwives' social recognition and legitimacy in the Italian context. Within the hospital, the role of the obstetrician and his interventions in the delivery room, even in cases of physiological pregnancies and births, is the most striking demonstration of an invasion of one profession by another. The medical (Freidson 1970; Tousijn 2000, 2004) and symbolic dominance (Bourdieu 1998) of obstetricians over midwives has diminished midwives' legitimacy as primary birth attendants, simultaneously transforming women's own perceptions of their bodies. As an emblem of the health and power of the female body, in modern patriarchal societies, childbirth must be rendered pathological to justify its domination by doctors (Duden 2006). Doulas, engaged in restoring to women the power of their own bodies and births, consider the midwife an ally and value her activity.

However, doulas' experiences with midwives can be ambivalent:

> … sometimes I have suffered great humiliations and mortifications from midwives. I was kicked out of a delivery room, treated badly … patience, I go on anyway … Once a midwife called me out and asked me: "Who gave you the permission to come with the mum?", I explained that there was no need for permission to accompany a mother and she: "No, no, I'm going to the head of the department now, I don't want you here with women". Obviously, nothing happened … another time … a couple of midwives asked me "what do you think of that labor?" especially one of them; she has always asked my opinion during a delivery, and they were very experienced people, older midwives.
>
> (Edda)

> … with a group of midwives who work in my area I had an experience of serene curiosity to understand and remove prejudices. Then I also had a negative experience with a midwife, of total denial or derision, almost as if to be a doula was a useless job … you are a freak, what do you do? Let's say these are the three ranges of reactions I have experienced: enthusiasm, curiosity, denial.
>
> (Dina)

> I have the good fortune to meet midwives who are friends of doulas, even here in the region where I work. With some of them it was a slow work of mutual knowledge, instead with some it was more love at first sight because they already knew exactly what I was doing. I also had big problems … I'll give you an example. I organized a meeting to inform mothers about different ways of delivering and I invited two hospital midwives and two freelance midwives, but their institutional bodies called the midwives involved when they heard about this meeting, they phoned each midwife to say "it's better you don't take part in a meeting organized by a doula" … a little mafia mode.
>
> (Elga)

When the delivery was over, I was leaving, and the midwife hugged me and said, "Thank you, thank you for your work" … Then I meet a young midwife who adores doulas ... but she said to me: "You know, we are educated at the university to hate you" ... I then believe that in the end the problem is just an abstract problem. When midwives know you, when they work with you, they understand that you are not what they think you are.

(Emma)

With these words, Emma indexes the solution to the midwife–doula split: midwives need exposure to doula care, so that their reactions to doulas are not based on gossip and innuendo, but rather on actual, embodied experience.

Also in doulas' representations, midwives appear as a fragmented group. Wide openings and availability of collaboration are flanked by denial or avoidance, in order to prevent potential retaliations by institutional representative bodies. This lack of internal cohesion and the opening up of certain professionals are decisive elements in the emergence of the doula profile, since it is in those interwoven fields' gray areas that the doula anchors part of her legitimacy. To overcome the resistances posed by some midwives, doulas have adopted a strategy that I define as an "omission of presentation":

I am bothered by the fact that, since my name is "doula," then midwives have preconceptions about me, to the point that I tried to organize informational meetings and events with a young midwife here in my town, and she asked me not to write on flyers that I am a doula, fearing rebukes from the national board.... I did it to protect her."

(Mara)

... in the pediatrician office or in the hospital ... if they don't ask me who I am, I won't say it.

(Susi)

Avoiding presenting themselves as doulas seems to be the most often adopted strategy. This "hiding" of the doulas' professional identity has the goal of avoiding possible tensions with the healthcare professionals who do not accept doulas and who could have a negative impact on the client. Moreover, by avoiding mentioning who they are, doulas try to protect collaborative midwives from the disciplinary rebukes that might stem from this collaboration.

In their practices, doulas appear to be eager to achieve substantial recognition by mothers and midwives. It is in starting from the bottom, from the valorization of personal relationships and the establishment of bonds of trust, that doulas anchor their legitimacy. The omission of the declaration of one's professional identity in certain circumstances serves to "prepare the ground" for the achievement of a wider cultural and social legitimacy. As previously noted, doulas tend to believe that once more midwives have worked with them, those midwives will spread the word about the benefits of doula practice, thereby opening up more cultural space for the development of mutually appreciative doula–midwife relationships and changing midwives' negative opinions about doulas.

Inter-professional relations

Previous sections have highlighted the different representations of midwives toward doulas, and vice versa. What has emerged as crucial is the split within the professional group of midwives: some contest doula practice, while others recognize doulas and desire to cooperate with them. In contrast to this midwifery disunity, doulas hold midwives in high regard and are willing and eager to increase midwife–doula collaborations. Adams (2007), expanding Abbott's (1988) model, which based professional development primarily on conflict, argues that in certain circumstances, professional development can take place through inter-professional cooperation and collaboration. The conditions for effective collaboration identified by Adams require a similarity in the size, outlook, and legislative status of the professional groups involved. In the case of doulas and midwives, it is possible to find only one of these conditions—albeit a powerful one: the similarity of outlook. Both professional groups strive for the well-being of mothers. This single element of affinity assumes a preponderant value, so much so as to push some midwives to cooperate with doulas, thereby contradicting the precepts of the National Federation of Midwives. If midwife–doula collaboration should increase, as some midwives wish, the coercive or intimidating methods of the National Midwife's Federation, which are already recognized as inappropriate by some members, risk causing an internal crisis. Thus, in order to avoid a confrontation among colleagues with unpredictable consequences, it is possible to imagine that eventually, the institutional representatives and all hospital midwives will agree to cooperate with doulas. In this sense, it is possible to hypothesize a scenario that simplifies the mutual affirmations of professions. If, within a professional group, some members are willing to cooperate with the neighboring group, animated by the sharing of a common outlook and fundamental values, the conditions for recognition and legitimacy of the formerly subordinated and stigmatized group will be created. Thus, I can imagine a national alliance of midwives and doulas that could raise the profiles of both professional groups, gain more autonomy for midwives, and cement their collaboration in maternity care.

The above is just one of the possible scenarios that could come to characterize and facilitate the development of the doula profession. A further development could involve the recognition of doulas by midwives in exchange for midwives' cognitive control of the birth process, which would include defining what the doula can or cannot do in the labor room.

For example, a few years ago, the association *Associazione Doule Italia* and the board of midwives in Milan got together to define the limits of doula practice and to outline the boundary between the two professions. However, the National Federation of Midwives has never approved this agreement, considering this action to be dangerous for the entire midwifery profession and so has effectively interrupted its development. Yet when national organizations fail to consider the desires of too many of their own members, those groups are likely to succumb to internal conflict and cease to exist in their current forms.

Finally, in imagining another possible development of the doula profession, it is useful to pay attention to the roles that doctors may play in this endeavor. The hospitalization of childbirth, the increasing medicalization of births, and the primary role acquired by obstetricians in assisting physiological pregnancy and childbirth could lead to a progressive weakening of the figure of the midwife. The tasks of the midwife could be acquired by nurses, since the clinical part would be managed completely by physicians. The managerialization of hospitals and the reduction of public funding for healthcare give plausibility to this hypothesis. In this case, doulas would find fertile ground for their development, since, on the one hand, emotional support for mothers would become their exclusive responsibility and, on the other hand, the hospital would welcome these people who would ease the burden on public resources. This is just a possible evolution of the dynamics and of course is not what doulas desire. What doulas do desire is to experience midwives as their allies in all contexts, and not their enemies. And should doulas and midwives become united, as suggested above, perhaps, in working together, they could help midwives to regain their professional jurisdiction over normal, physiological birth, reserving obstetricians for the pathologies with which they are trained to assist. As has been demonstrated in New Zealand (Georges and Daellenbach 2019) and the Netherlands (Cheyney et al. 2019), the appropriate, evidence-based ratio for birth attendance is midwives: 80% and obstetricians: 20%. This ratio, especially when combined with doula assistance during labor and birth, has been shown to produce the most optimal outcomes for mothers and newborns.

Conclusion

In this chapter, I have highlighted midwives' both negative and positive representations of doulas and doulas' generally positive representations of midwives, in order to get at the underpinnings of their inter-professional conflicts and cooperations. My takeaway impression is that doulas will be able to develop fruitful inter-professional relations with midwives who are open to working with doulas, and thus gradually, the opposition to doulas currently perpetrated by the National Federation of Midwives and by hospital midwives will lose its relevance, since doulas will be able to specify and communicate more effectively about the nature and focus of their profession, thereby negating the reasons for that opposition.

My research has shown that midwives' representations of doulas are often confused, vague, and not relevant to what the doula actually does. In other words, the conflict with midwives has allowed doulas to accurately define their cultural jurisdiction, to perfect the communication strategies they use to describe that jurisdiction, and to focus on building a social structure capable of defending their profession in the legal, public opinion, and workplace arenas. In this sense, I can extend Abbott's theorization (1988) by considering that the conflict between these two professions has made it possible for doulas to clarify and specify their areas of expertise and jurisdiction, and to make it clear how these differ from those of midwives. This specification could ultimately remove the reasons for the doula–midwife conflict. For Italian midwives and doulas, it doesn't have to be "either-or"; rather, it can be "both-and"—if they join together to work collaboratively in what Jordan (1983) called "mutual accommodation."

Conclusion

In this book, I have explored the profession of the doula, with particular focus on Italian doulas. To recap, the doula profile began to develop in the U.S.A. in the 1980s, and now doulas are present worldwide. In Italy, doulas started their development in the early 2000s. By this time of writing (September 2021), around 1000 Italian doulas have been trained, and it is possible to estimate, as reported by the presidents of the main doula associations, that about half of those trained are in active practice as professional doulas. Doulas' activities are legitimized by Law Number 4 of 2013.

To date, there are no data on the percentage of Italian births attended by doulas. Anecdotal reports from doula interlocutors show that this percentage is still quite small, as Italian childbearers are only recently learning about the many benefits of doula care. Doulas are allowed by the main doula associations to attend births only together with midwives or obstetricians. Yet despite this official restriction, some few doulas who are not members of any doula associations do attend "unassisted births"—those with no biomedical practitioners present. The majority of Italian doulas consider this behavior risky for mothers and babies and for doulas' professionalization process. I have investigated the process through which these care providers are affirming their cultural and social jurisdictions through the study of doula training courses, practices implemented, and intra- and interprofessional relationships.

The doula profession in Italy: from illusory inconsistency to patchwork consistency

To support childbearing women throughout the perinatal process, doulas embody and employ a pluralism of symbols, meanings, and systems of knowledge. The doula is a social care profession that I have named *doulaing*, which can be described with the metaphor of patchwork. What gives coherence to this patchwork are the particular texture and designs into which the differing elements are assembled. Doula work is designed around a specific relational style and a set of skills that work to facilitate and enhance the perinatal experience. This expertise and relational style give consistency

DOI: 10.4324/9781003165934-8

to the patchwork. To understand the doula profession in Italy, I find it useful to imagine a large patchwork quilt of many colors, in which each small quilt piece is created by an individual doula. Together these quilting pieces, when sewn together, create a larger, recognizably coherent pattern. And I like to think of this quilt as a blanket available to all childbearers to warm, comfort, protect, and empower them in the multiple, patchworks ways that doulas employ.

Therefore, I wondered about the possibility for such a pluralistic profile to affirm and legitimize its own cultural jurisdiction. The answer was found in their various practices and techniques. Dynamism, flexibility, and personalization of care characterize the work of the doula. This is how these professionals can assemble, interlink, and mix different elements of knowledge and experience, depending on the client. Their flexible practices allow the integration of multiple cultural elements. Doulas learn this flexibility by treating each other as they treat their clients.

Patchwork is emblematic

The metaphor of patchwork has been used by Balbo (2008) to describe women's ways of working and living in everyday life, yet patchwork also represents strategies and moments of gratification and pleasure. The practice of patchwork can open the ability to gradually adapt the design, the project, without preestablished models and capturing the specificity of what is needed at the moment. Considering the uniqueness of each individual experience of pregnancy and childbirth, and given the contemporary cultural pluralism in Italy, to develop the work of the doula, it is necessary to have a wide and diversified range of resources to draw from in order to offer individualized support. The expertise of these professionals lies mainly in the ways in which doulas offer their skills to clients, according to a specific style of relationship. This expertise gives consistency to the patchwork.

Parallel to the definition of cultural jurisdiction, the Italian doula profession is engaged in the creation of a social structure able to guarantee its effectiveness toward crucial audiences: the state/legal system, public opinion, and the workplace. Doulas have developed the process of legitimizing their profession in these arenas in various ways. In the public opinion arena, doulas have reached a good level of recognition, while, in the workplace arena, partial recognition has been achieved, since the doula is only partially legitimized among maternity care professionals. And in the state/legal arena, the process is ongoing. Considering the rapid evolution in the Italian context, it is likely that doulas will develop strategies to achieve legal recognition, according to the provisions of Law 4/2013, and that this will promote the legitimacy of the doula among other maternity care professionals. Cultural jurisdiction will act as guarantor of social jurisdiction.

During the postpartum period, the Italian doulas support the mother and the family, combining in a single figure tasks and roles that used to be covered by family members, such as cooking and babysitting. Doulas work to satisfy clients' needs and to stimulate a reflective process, both for their clients and for themselves. Attention to the doula–mother relationship, and to the fact that everyone has a voice, and that this voice needs to be heard and understood, are the ethics that characterize doula care work. Care is for doulas both a process and a practice, involving both action and reflection. It encompasses particular attention to relational styles and to listening to women in the typical ways performed by doulas, which are opposed to the absence of real listening that women denounce, based on their experiences in hospitals, clinics, and other biomedical care contexts. Medical excess finds expression in the standardization of medical procedures, in the prevalent and often unnecessary use of diagnostic and interventive technologies, and in the objectification and pathologization of pregnancy and childbirth. Pregnant or new mothers turn to doulas to accomplish a return to subjectivity and self-determination.

The meanings that doulas give to their profession can differ, and thus, I have identified three doula types: the progressive doula, the philanthropic doula, and the individualistic doula. To recap, the progressive doula gives her activity a political–cultural meaning. The aim of this type of doula is to activate empowerment processes, so that women can make decisions regarding pregnancy and childbirth without the oppression that the biomedical system perpetrates. Therefore, the progressive doula aspires to a cultural change that the transformative potential of pregnancy and childbirth can facilitate. The philanthropic doula considers her own practice as a mission and a vocation, and the meanings she gives to it are social and humanistic. The objective of her doula work is to help women and families to deal gracefully with this delicate period. The individualistic doula attributes personal meaning to her practice, thinking of it as a lifestyle. Although there are differences among them, what unites individualistic doulas is an eclectic attitude and an accentuated individual charisma, which elevates them either to a model to follow or to the opposite—a model that should not be practiced by other doulas.

Yet despite the different meanings that doulas attribute to their practices and holding different values and perspectives, the professional group maintains a public face of unity, thanks to their embodiment of a rhetoric of sisterhood and solidarity able to provide cohesion and consistency among the patchwork of doula organizations and practices. The ability of Italian doulas to adopt a strategy that gives a lower value to the divergent elements and a higher value to the convergent elements, and the shared adoption of this specific rhetoric, represent the keys to ensuring the ongoing development of the professional doula in Italy and to ensuring that Italian doulas will not become mired in infighting but will present a relatively united front to the government and the public.

The history of a profession must be contextualized within the wider history of the system of professions (Abbott 2010). Midwives constitute the professional group closest to doulas. As I have shown throughout this book, the National Federation of Midwives has opposed doulas since their beginning. However, the group of midwives is not homogeneous on this issue: whereas the larger part of the professional group opposes doulas, the rest recognize them and the value of the services they provide and are willing to cooperate with them. For their part, doulas are cohesive in their desire to develop alliances with midwives. Both professional groups aspire to the well-being of childbearers; this shared goal takes on a preponderant value, such as to encourage some midwives to collaborate with doulas even when facing rebukes from their institutional board. The possibility of collaboration between Italian midwives and doulas could represent an important development for mothers, who stand to benefit most from such a collaboration. In this way, both professional groups will see their main professional objective reached.

The study of the doula also calls for a further reflection that includes the biomedical field, and in particular a possible tendency to reassess the doctor–patient relationship. Increasingly informed women will show more and more awareness about their birth choices, urging a transformation in the dialogical sense of their relationships with healthcare providers. The revaluation and enhancement of the relationship between doctor and patient not only will stimulate greater confidence and satisfaction among patients but may also have positive effects by reducing the costs of maternity care, since through dialogue facilitated by doulas, many diagnostic examinations and the practice of defensive medicine will become unnecessary. Fielding (1990) noted that doctors are under opposing pressures: on the one hand, there are reforms to control health spending; on the other hand, the change in consumer–patient behavior leads doctors—especially obstetricians—to practice defensive medicine, which is responsible for producing an increase in maternity care costs. The key to overcoming this tension lies, in my opinion, in the abandonment of defensive medicine as a practice and in the enhancement of the doctor–patient relationship, which can be greatly aided by doulas. In other words, what the doula profession urges to the biomedical maternity care professions is a paradigm shift. The biomedical paradigm must give way to a social–humanistic paradigm that requires the revaluation of relationships and the identification of times, spaces, and procedures that assure to the pregnant and birthgiving mother, who is in one of the moments of the maximum creative power of life, that she will be seen, heard, and touched—behaviors that are practiced and thus modeled by doulas.

Bibliography

Abbott A., (1988), *The System of Professions. An Essay on the Division of Expert Labor*, The University of Chicago Press, Chicago, IL.

Abbott A., (1991), The Future of Professions: Occupations and Expertise on the Age of Organization, *Research in the Sociology of Organizations*, 8 (1):17–42.

Abbott A., (2010), Varieties of Ignorance, *The American Sociologist*, 41 (2):174–189.

Abbott A., (2014), The Problem of Excess, *Sociological Theory*, 32 (1):1–26. DOI: 10.1177/0735275114523419.

Abbott A., (2018), *Lezioni italiane*, Orthotes Editrice, Napoli-Salerno.

Abramson R., Breedlove G., Isaacs B., (2006), *The Community-Based Doula: Supporting Families Before, During, and After Childbirth*, Zero to Three Press, Washington, DC.

Adams T.L., (2007), Inter-Professional Relations and the Emergence of a New Profession: Software Engineering in Canada, the US and the UK, *The Sociological Quarterly*, 48 (3):507–532.

Adams T.L., (2015), Sociology of Professions: International Divergences and Research Directions, *Work, Employment and Society*, 29 (1):154–165. DOI: 10.1177/0950017014523467.

Adler P.A., Adler P., (1987), *Membership Roles in Field Research*, Sage, Thousand Oaks, CA.

Akhavan, S., Lundgren, I., (2012), Midwives' Experiences of Doula Support for Immigrant Women in Sweden – A Qualitative Study, *Midwifery*, 28 (1):80–85.

Albert M., (1991), *Capitalism against Capitalism*, Whurr Publishers, London.

Anderson G.M., (2004), Making Sense of Rising Cesarean Section Rates, *British Medical Journal*, 329:696–697.

Asselin M.E., (2003), Insider Research. Issues to Consider When Doing Qualitative Research in Your Own Setting, *Journal for Nurses in Staff Development*, 19 (2):99–103.

Balbo L., (2008), *Il lavoro e la cura*, Einaudi, Torino.

Ballard K., Elston M.A., (2005), Medicalisation. A Multi-Dimensional Concept, *Social Theory and Health*, 3:228–241.

Barley S.R., Kunda G., (2004), *Gurus, Hired Guns and Warm Body*, Princeton University Press, Princeton, NJ.

Basile M.R., (2012), *Reproductive Justice and Childbirth Reform: Doulas as Agent of Social Change*, PhD dissertation, University of Iowa.

Basile M.R., (2015), Reimagining the Birthing Body. Reproductive Justice and New Directions in Doula Care, in Castañeda A.N., Johnson Searcy J., (eds.), *Doulas and Intimate Labour. Boundaries, Bodies, and Birth*, Demeter Press, Bradford, ON.

Basmajian A., (2014), Abortion Doulas. Changing the Narrative, *Anthropology Now*, 6 (2):44–51.

Bauman Z., (2007), *Consuming Life*, Polity Press, Cambridge.

Benaglia B., (2018), "Mothering the Mother": Doulas and the Affective Space, in Lane J., Joensusu E., (eds.), *Everyday World-Making: Toward an Understanding of Affect and Mothering*, Demeter Press, Bradford, ON.

Benaglia B., (2020), La cura invisibile: potenzialità e limiti della pratica della doula, *Antropologia e teatro*, 12:59–83. https://doi.org/10.6092/issn.2039-2281/10885.

Benaglia B., (2022), *Lo spazio della doula. Pratiche di cura e accompagnamento alla maternità*, Meltemi, Milano.

Beoku-Betts J., (1994), When Black Is Not Enough. Doing Field Research among Gullah Women, *NWSA Journal*, 6 (3):413–433.

Berg M., Terstad A., (2006), Swedish Women's Experiences of Doula Support During Childbirth, *Midwifery*, 22 (4):330–338.

Bertaux D., (1999), *Racconti di vita. La prospettiva etnosociologica*, Franco Angeli, Milano.

Bertolo C., (2013), *Soggettività e yoga. Prime riflessioni da una ricerca*, Unipress, Padova.

Bestetti G., Colombo G., Regalia A., (2005), *Mani sul parto, mani nel parto. Mantenere normale la nascita*, Carocci, Roma.Betran A.P., Torloni M.R., Zhang J., Ye J., Mikolajczyk R., Deneux-Tharaux C., Oladapo O.T., Souza J.P., Tunçalp O., Vogel J.P., Gülmezoglu A.M., (2015), What Is the Optimal Rate of Caesarean Section at Population Level? A Systematic Review of Ecologic Studies, *Reproductive Health*, 12 (57):1–10. DOI: 10.1186/s12978-015-0043-6.

Bettini M., (1998), *Nascere. Storie di donne, donnole, madri ed eroi*, Einaudi, Torino.

Bimbi F., (1995), Etica della cura. Stili di vita adulta e organizzazione, *Animazione Sociale*, 2:9–15.

Bimbi F., (2000), Se lo specialismo nega l'ascolto, *Animazione Sociale*, 141:3–10.

Blackford H., (2005), The Wandering Womb at Home in the Red Tent. An Adolescent Bildungsroman in a Different Voice, *The ALAN Review*, 32 (2):74–85.

Bohren M.A, Berger B.O., Munthe-Kaas H., Tunçalp O., (2019), Perceptions and Experiences of Labour Companionship: A Qualitative Evidence Synthesis, *Cochrane Database Systematic Review*, 18, 3 (3):CD012449. DOI: 10.1002/14651858.CD012449.pub2.

Bourdieu P., (1998), *Il dominio maschile*, Feltrinelli, Milano.

Bourgeault, I., Benoit C., Davis-Floyd R., (eds.), (2004), *Reconceiving Midwifery*, McGill-Queens University Press, Montreal.

Breedlove G., (2005), Perceptions of Social Support from Pregnant and Parenting Teens Using Community-Based Doulas, *Journal of Perinatal Education*, 14:15–22.

Bruni A., Gheradi S., (2007), *Studiare le pratiche lavorative*, Il Mulino, Bologna.

Burkitt I., (2012), Emotional Reflexivity. Feeling, Emotion and Imagination in Reflexive Dialogues, *Sociology*, 46 (3):458–472.

Burrage M., (1990), Introduction. The Professions in Sociology and History, in Torstendahl R., Burrage M., (eds.), *The Formation of Professions. Knowledge, State and Strategy*, Sage, London.Campbell D.A., Lake M.F., Falk M., Backstrand J.F., (2006), A Randomized Control Trial of Continuous Support in Labor by a Lay Doula, *Journal of Obstetric, Gynecologic, & Neonatal Nursing*, 35 (4):456–464.

Campbell D., Scott K.D., Klaus M.H., Falk M., (2007), Female Relatives or Friends Trained as Labor Doulas: Outcomes at 6 to 8 Weeks Postpartum, *Birth*, 34:220–227.

Campero L., Garcia C., Diaz C., Ortiz O., Reynoso S., Langer A., (1998), "Alone, I Wouldn't Have Known What to Do". A Qualitative Study on Social Support during Labor and Delivery in Mexico, *Social Science and Medicine*, 47 (3):395–403.

Carr-Saunders A.P., Wilson P.A., (1933), *The Professions*, Oxford University Press, Oxford.

Castañeda A.N., Searcy J.J., (eds.), (2015), *Doulas and Intimate Labour: Boundaries, Bodies, and Birth*, Demeter Press, Bradford, ON.

Castel R., (2009), *La montée des inceritudes. Travail, protections, statut de l'individu*, Editions du Seuil, Paris.

Chen C.C, Lee J.F., (2020), Effectiveness of the Doula Program in Northern Taiwan, *Tzu Chi Medical Journal*, 32 (4):373–379.

Cheyney M., (2011), Reinscribing the Birthing Body: Homebirth as Ritual Performance, *Medical Anthropology Quarterly*, 25 (4):519–542. DOI: 10.1111/j.1548-1387.2011.01183.x.

Cheyney M., Bahareh G., Therese W., Davis-Floyd R., and Saraswathi V., (2019), Giving Birth in the United States and the Netherlands: Midwifery Care as Integrated Option or Contested Privilege?, in Davis-Floyd R., Cheyney M., (eds.), *Birth in Eight Cultures*, Long Waveland Press, Grove, IL.

Cheyney M., Davis-Floyd R., (2020a), Birth and the Big Bad Wolf: A Biocultural, Co-Evolutionary Perspective, Part 1, *International Journal of Childbirth*, 9 (4):177–192. DOI: 10.1891/IJCBIRTH-D-19-00030.

Cheyney M., Davis-Floyd R., (2020b), Birth and the Big Bad Wolf: A Biocultural, Co-Evolutionary Perspective, Part 2, *International Journal of Childbirth*, 10 (2):66–78. DOI: 10.1891/IJCBIRTH-D-19-00029.

Cheyney M., Davis-Floyd R., (2021), Birth and the Big Bad Wolf: Biocultural Evolution and Human Childbirth, in Davis Floyd R., (ed.), *Birthing Techno-Sapiens: Human-Technology Co-Evolution and the Future of Reproduction*, Routledge, Abingdon.

Chor J., Hill B., Martins S., Mistretta S., Patel A., Gilliam M., (2015), Doula Support during First-Trimester Surgical Abortion. A Randomized Controlled Trial, *American Journal of Obstetrics & Gynecology*, 212 (45):1–6.

Christiaens W., Bracke P., (2007), Assessment of Social Psychological Determinants of Satisfaction with Childbirth in a Cross-National Perspective, *BMC Pregnancy and Childbirth*, 7 (26). https://doi.org/10.1186/1471-2393-7-26.

Collins R., (1990), Changing Conceptions in the Sociology of Professions, in Torstendahl R., Burrage M., (eds.), *The Formation of Professions. Knowledge, State and Strategy*, Sage, London.

Colombo E., (2003), Trasformazioni sociali e nuovi modi di pensare la salute e la malattia, in Colombo E., Rebughini P., (eds.), *La medicina che cambia. Le terapie non convenzionali in Italia*, il Mulino, Bologna.Colombo G., (2004), *Cura, lavoro di cura, relazione: parole, immagini e concetti in evoluzione*, in Colombo G., Cocever E., Bianchi L., (eds.), *Il lavoro di cura*, Carocci, Roma.

Colombo G., Pizzini F., Regalia A., (1985), *Mettere al mondo. La produzione sociale del parto*, Franco Angeli, Milano.

Colombo E., Rebughini P., (eds.), (2003), *La medicina che cambia. Le terapie non convenzionali in Italia*, il Mulino, Bologna.

Conrad P., (1992), Medicalization and Social Control, *Annual Review of Sociology*, 18:209–232.

Corbin Dwyer S., Buckle J.L., (2009), The Space Between. On Being an Insider-Outsider in Qualitative Research, *International Journal of Qualitative Methods*, 8 (1):54–63.

Corsaro W., (1985), *Friendship and Peer Culture in the Early Years*, Ablex Publishing Corporation, Norwood, NJ.

Cortlund Y., Lucke B., Miller Watelet D., (2006), *Mother Rising. The Blessingway Journey into Motherhood*, Celestial Arts, Berkeley, CA.

Coyle C.W., Hulse K.E., Wisner K.L., Driscoll K.E., Clark C.T., (2015), Placentophagy: Therapeutic Miracle or Myth?, *Archives Women's Mental Health*, 18 (5):673–680.

Curi U., (2012), Uniti da un confine, *Corriere della Sera*. 16/12/2012.

Dal Lago A., (2004), *Non-persone. L'esclusione dei migranti in una società globale*, Feltrinelli, Milano.

Davis-Floyd R., (1994), The Technocratic Body. American Childbirth as Cultural Expression, *Social Science e Medicine*, 38:1125–1140.

Davis-Floyd R., (2001), The Technocratic, Humanistic, and Holistic Paradigms of Childbirth, *International Journal of Gynecology and Obstetrics*, 75:5–23.

Davis-Floyd R., (2018), *Ways of Knowing about Birth. Mothers, Midwives, Medicine, and Birth Activism*, Waveland Press, Long Grove, IL.

Davis-Floyd R., (2003, 2022) *Birth as an American Rite of Passage*, Routledge, Abingdon.

Davis-Floyd R., Gutschow K., Schwartz D.A., (2020), Pregnancy, Birth, and the COVID-19 Pandemic in the United States, *Medical Anthropology*, 39 (5):413–427. DOI: 10.1080/01459740.2020.1761804.

Davis-Floyd R., Johnson, C.B., (eds.), (2006), *Mainstreaming Midwives: The Politics of Change*, Routledge, New York, NY.

Davis-Floyd R., Laughlin C.D., (2022), *Ritual: What It Is, How It Works, and Why*, Berghahn Books, New York, NY.

Davis-Floyd R., Matsuoka E., Horan H., Ruder B., Everson C.L., (2018), Daughter of Time: The Postmodern Midwife, in Davis-Floyd R., (ed.), *Ways of Knowing about Birth: Mothers, Midwives, Medicine, and Birth Activism*, Waveland Press, Long Gove, IL.

Davis-Floyd R., Sargent C.F., (1997), *Childbirth and Authoritative Knowledge. Cross-Cultural Perspectives*, University of California Press, Berkley, CA.

Deitrick L.M., Draves P.R., (2008), Attitudes towards Doula Support during Pregnancy by Clients, Doulas, and Labor-and-Delivery Nurses: A Case Study from Tampa, Florida, *Human Organization*, 67 (4):397–406.

Denzin N.K., (1984), *On Understanding Emotion*, Jossey-Bass, San Francisco, CA.

De Vries R., Benoit C., van Teijlingen E., Wrede S., (eds.), (2001), *Birth by Design: Pregnancy, Maternity Care and Midwifery in North America and Europe*, Routledge, London.

Diamant A., (1997), *The Red Tent*, St. Martin's Press, New York, NY.

Duden B., (1991), *Il corpo della donna come luogo pubblico. Sull'abuso del concetto di vita*, Bollati Boringhieri, Torino.

Duden B., (2006), *I geni in testa e il feto nel grembo*, Bollati Boringhieri, Torino.

Earp J.A.L., French E.A., Gilkey M.B., (2008), *Patient Advocacy for Health Care Quality. Strategies for Achieving Patient-Centered Care*, Jones and Bartlett, Sudbury, MA.

Ehrenreich B., English D., (1977), *Le streghe siamo noi. Il ruolo della medicina nella repressione della donna*, La salamandra, Milano.

Elias N., (2007), *The Genesis of the Naval Profession*, University College Dublin Press, Dublin.

Ellis C., (1995), *Final Negotiations. A Story of Love, Loss and Chronic Illness*, Temple University Press, Philadelphia, PA.

Ellis C., Adams T., Bochner A., (2011), Autoethnography. An Overview, *Historical Social Research*, 36 (4):273–290.

Emerson J.P., (2008), Behaviour in Private Places: Sustaining Definitions of Reality in Gynecological Examinations, *Recent Sociology*, 74 (2):74–97.

Etzioni A., (1970), *The Semi-Professions and Their Organization: Teachers, Nurses, Social Workers, New York*, The Free Press, New York, NY.

Evetts J., (2003), The Sociological Analysis of Professionalism. Occupational Change in the Modern World, *International Sociology*, 18 (2):295–416.

Evetts J., (2008), Introduction: Professional Work in Europe. Concepts, Theories, and Methodologies, *European Societies*, 10 (4):525–544.

Fielding S.L., (1990), Physician Reactions to Malpractice Suits and Cost Containment in Massachusetts, *Work and Occupations*, 17 (3):302–319.

Filippini N.M., (1995), *La nascita straordinaria. Tra madre e figlio la rivoluzione del taglio cesareo (sec. XVIII-XIX)*, Franco Angeli, Milano.

Filippini N.M., (2017), *Generare, partorire, nascere. Una storia dall'antichità alla provetta*, Viella, Roma.

Flamm B.L., Berwick D.M., Kabcenell A., (1998), Reducing Cesarean Section Rates Safely: Lessons from a 'Breakthrough Series' Collaborative, *Birth*, 25:117–124.

Freidson E., (1970), *Professional Dominance. The Social Structure of Medical Care*, Atheron, New York, NY.

Freidson E., (2001), *Professionalism. The Third Logic*, University of Chicago Press, Chicago, IL.

Freire P., (1970/ 2006), *Pedagogy of the Oppressed: 30th Anniversary Edition*, Continuum, New York, NY.

Fisher J., Astbury J., Smith A., (1997), Adverse Psychological Impact of Operative Obstetric Interventions. A Perspective Longitudinal Study, *Australian and New Zealand Journal of Psychiatry*, 31:728–738.

Fox B., Worts D., (1999), Revisiting the Critique of Medicalized Childbirth: A Contribution to the Sociology of Birth, *Gender and Society*, 13 (3):326–346.

Gallino L., (2003), *La scomparsa dell'Italia industriale*, Einaudi Editore, Torino.

Gaskin I.M., (2003), *La gioia del parto. Segreti e virtù del corpo femminile durante il travaglio e la nascita*, Bonomi Editore, Pavia.

Gazzaniga V., (2014), *La medicina antica*, Carocci Editore, Roma.

Gentry Q.M., Nolte K.M., Gonzalez A., Pearson M., Ivey S., (2010), "Going beyond the Call of Doula": A Grounded Theory Analysis of the Diverse Roles Community-Based Doulas Play in the Lives of Pregnant and Parenting Adolescent Mothers, *Journal of Perinatal Education*, 19:24–40.

George, M., (2013), Seeking Legitimacy: The Professionalization of Life Coaching, *Sociological Inquiry*, 83 (2):179–208.

Georges E., Daellenbach R., (2019), Divergent Meanings and Practices of Childbirth in Greece and New Zealand, in Davis-Floyd R., Cheyney M., (eds.), *Birth in Eight Cultures*, Waveland Press, Long Grove, IL.

Giacomini M., (1992), Scene del parto e ordini simbolici. Storia di un conflitto perdurante, in Sbisà M., (ed.), *Come sapere il parto*, Rosenberg & Sellier, Torino.

Gilligan C., (1982), *Con voce di donna. Etica e formazione della personalità*, Feltrinelli, Milano.Gilliland A., (2002), Beyond Holding Hands: The Modern Role of the Professional Doula, *Journal of Obstetric, Gynecologic, and Neonatal Nursing*, 31 (6):762–769.

Gilliland A., (2010), *A Grounded Theory Model of Effective Labor Support By Doulas*, PhD Dissertation in Philosophy, University of Wisconsin-Madison.

Gobo G., (2001), *Descrivere il mondo. Teoria e pratica del metodo etnografico in sociologia*, Carocci, Roma.

Goer H., (1995), *Obstetric Myths versus Research Realities*, Bergin and Garvey Publishers, New York, NY.

Gordon N.P., Walton D., McAdam E., Derman J., Gallitero G., Garrett L., (1999), Effects of Providing Hospital-Based Doulas in Health Maintenance Organization Hospitals, *Obstetrics and Gynecology*, 93:422–426.

Greenwood E., (1957), Attributes of a Profession, *Social Work*, II (3):44–55.

He M., (2011), *Doulas Going Dutch: The Role of Professional Labor Support in the Netherlands*, Rice University, Independent Study Project (ISP) Collection. http://digitalcollections.sit.edu/isp_collection/1153/.

Henley M.M., (2015), Alternative and Authoritative Knowledge: The Role of Certification for Defining Expertise among Doulas, *Social Currents*, 2 (3):260–279.

Henley M.M., (2016), *Science and Service. Doula Work and the Legitimacy of Alternative Knowledge System*, PhD Dissertation in Sociology, University of Arizona.

Henrion R., (2008), Les doulas: une profession émergente?, *Bulletin de l'Academie Nationale de Medecine*, 192 (6):1237–1252.

Hodnett E.D., (1999), *Caregiver Support for Women During Childbirth*, Cochrane Library, Oxford.

Hodnett E.D., Gates S., Hofmeyr G.J., Sakala C., (2013), Continuous Support for Women during Childbirth (Review), *Cochrane Database of Systematic Reviews*, 7:1–114.

Hofmeyr J.G., Nikodem C.V., Wolman W.L., Chalmers B.E., Kramer T., (1991), Companionship to Modify the Clinical Birth Environment: Effects on Progress and Perceptions of Labour, and Breastfeeding, *British Journal of Obstetrics and Gynecology*, 98:756–764.

Holmes M., (2010), The Emotionalization of Reflexivity, *Sociology*, 44 (1):139–154.

Holmes M., (2015), Researching Emotional Reflexivity, *Emotion Review*, 7 (1):61–66.

Hughes E.C., (1958), *Men and Their Work*, Free Press, New York, NY.

Hundley V.A., Milne J.M., Glazener C.M.A., Mollison J., (1997), Satisfaction and the Three C's: Continuity, Choice and Control. Women's View from a Randomized Controlled Trial of Midwife-Led Care, *British Journal of Obstetrics and Gynaecology*, 104:1273–1280.

Illich I., (1976), *Limits to Medicine. Medical Nemesis: The Expropriation of Health*, Marion Boyars, London.

Ireland S., Montgomery-Andersen R., Geraghtya S., (2019), Indigenous Doulas: A Literature Review Exploring Their Role and Practice in Western Maternity Care, *Midwifery*, 75:52–58.

Istat, (2018), *Gravidanza, Parto e Allattamento al seno*, Roma. https://www.istat.it/it/archivio/141431.

Jedlowski P., (1986), *Il tempo dell'esperienza*, Franco Angeli, Milano.Johanson R., Newburn M., Macfarlane A., (2002), Has the Medicalization of Childbirth Gone too Far?, *British Medical Journal*, 324:892–895.

Johnson T.J., (1972), *Professions and Power*, MacMillan, London.

Jordan B., (1983), *Birth in Four Cultures*, Eden Press, London.

Kanuha V.L., (2000), "Being" Native versus "Going Native". Conducting Social Work Research as an Insider, *Social Work*, 45 (5):439–447.

Kayne M.A., Greulich M.B., Albers L.L., (2001), Doulas: An Alternative Yet Complementary Addition to Care during Childbirth, *Clinical Obstetrics and Gynecology*, 44 (4):692–703.

Kennell J., Klaus M., McGrath S., Robertson S., Hinkley C., (1991), Continuous Emotional Support during Labor in a US Hospital. A Randomized Controlled Trial, *JAMA—The Journal of the American Medical Association*, 265 (17):197–201.

Kittay E.F., (1999), *Love's Labor. Essay on Women, Equality, and Dependency*, Routledge, New York, NY.

Kittay E.F., (2001), A Feminist Public Ethic of Care Meets the New Communitarian Family Policy, *Ethics*, 111 (3):523–547.

Klaus M.H., Kennell J.H., (1983), *Bonding: The Beginnings of Parent-Infant Attachment*, C.V. Mosby Company, St. Louis, MO.

Klaus M.H., Kennell J.H., Klaus P.H., (1993), *Mothering the Mother. How a Doula Can Help You Have a Shorter, Easier and Healthier Birth*, Addison-Wesley Publishing Company, Menlo Park, CA.

Klaus M., Kennell J., Robertson S., Sosa R., (1986), Effects of Social Support during Parturition on Maternal and Infant Morbidity, *British Medical Journal*, 293:585–587.

Kornelson J., Grzybowski S., (2005), Safety and Community: The Maternity Care Needs of Rural Parturient Women, *Journal of Obstetrics and Gynaecology Canada*, 27 (6):554–561.

Kozhimannil K.B., Hardeman R.R., Alarid-Escudero F., Vogelsang C.A., Blauer-Peterson C., Howell E.A., (2016), Modeling the Cost-Effectiveness of Doula Care Associated with Reductions in Preterm Birth and Cesarean Delivery, *Birth*, 43 (1):20–27.

Krawczyk M., Rush M., (2020), *Describing the End-of-Life Doula Role and Practices of Care: Perspectives from Four Countries, Palliative Care & Social Practice*, 14:1–15.

La Mendola S., (2009), *Centrato e aperto. Dare vita a interviste dialogiche*, UTET, Torino.

La Rosa M., (2005), Immateriale, produzione, lavoro, *Sociologia del lavoro*, 99:25–30.

Lazarus E.S., (1994), What Do Women Want. Issues of Choice, Control, and Class in Pregnancy and Childbirth, *Medical Anthropology Quarterly*, 8:25–46.

Leboyer F., (1974), *Per una nascita senza violenza*, Bompiani, Milano.

Lim R.I., (2015), *Placenta. The Forgotten Chakra*, Half Angel Press, Bali.

Lombardi L., Pizzini F., (2004), La costruzione sociale del corpo femminile, in AA.VV., (eds.), *Un'appropriazione indebita*, Baldini e Castoldi, Milano.

Lowenberg J.S., Davis F., (1994), Beyond Medicalization-Demedicalisation. The Case of Holistic Health, *Sociology of Health and Illness*, 16:579–599.

Maestripieri L., (2013), *Consulenti di management. Il professionalismo organizzativo nel lavoro della conoscenza*, L'Harmattan Italia, Torino.

Mahoney M., Mitchell L., (2016), *The Doulas. Radical Care for Pregnant Women*, Feminist Press, New York, NY.

Maluccelli L., (2007), *Lavori di cura. Cooperazione sociale e servizi alla persona. L'esperienza di Cadiai*, Il Mulino, Bologna.

Manning-Orenstein G., (1998), A Birth Intervention: The Therapeutic Effects of Doula Support versus Lamaze Preparation on First-Time Mothers' Working Models of Caregiving, *Alternative Therapies in Health and Medicine*, 4 (4):73–81.

Mansfield B., (2008), The Social Nature of Natural Childbirth, *Social Science and Medicine*, 66:1084–1094.

Martin E., (2001), *The Woman in the Body. A Cultural Analysis of Reproduction*, Beacon Press, Boston, MA.

Maturo A., Conrad P., (eds.), (2009), *La medicalizzazione della vita, Salute e Società*, 2, Franco Angeli, Milano.

McClelland C.E., (1990), Escape from Freedom? Reflections on German Professionalization 1870-1933, in Torstendahl R., Burrage M., (eds.), *The Formation of Professions. Knowledge, State and Strategy*, Sage, London.

McComish J.F., Visger, J.M., (2009), Domains of Post-Partum Doula Care and Maternal Responsiveness and Competence, *Journal of Obstetric, Gynecologic, and Neonatal Nursing*, 38 (2):148–156.

McGrath S., Kennell J., (2008), A Randomized Controlled Trial of Continuous Labor Support for Middle-Class Couples. Effect on Cesarean Delivery Rates, *Birth*, 35 (2): 92–97.

Meltzer B., (2004), *Paid Labor: Labor Support Doulas and the Institutional Control of Birth*, PhD Dissertation, University of Pennsylvania.

Melucci A., (1998), *Verso una sociologia riflessiva*, Il Mulino, Bologna.

Merchant C., (1988), *La morte della natura. Le donne, l'ecologia e la rivoluzione scientifica*, Garzanti, Milano.

Merriam S.B., Johnson-Bailey J., Lee M-Y., Kee Y., Ntseane G., Muhamad M., (2001), Power and Positionality: Negotiating Insider/Outsider Status within and across Cultures, *International Journal of Lifelong Education*, 20 (5):405–416.

Merton R., (1972), Insiders and Outsiders. A Chapter in the Sociology of Knowledge, *American Journal of Sociology*, 78 (1):9–47.

Miller S., Abalos E., Chamillard M., Ciapponi A., Colaci D., Comandé D., Diaz V., Geller S., Hanson C., Langer A., Manuelli V., Millar K., Morhason-Bello I., Castro C.P., Pileggi V.N., Robinson N., Skaer M., Souza J.P., Vogel J.P., Althabe F., (2016), Beyond too Little, too Late and too Much, too Soon: A Pathway towards Evidence-Based, Respectful Maternity Care Worldwide, *Lancet*, 388 (10056):2176–2192. DOI: 10.1016/S0140-6736(16)31472-6.

Millerson G., (1964), *The Qualifying Associations*, Routledge, London.

Mills C.W., (1959), *The Sociological Imagination*, Oxford University Press, Oxford.

Minicuci M., (1985), Nascere e partorire tra presente e passato, in Oakley A., (ed.), *Le culture del parto*, Feltrinelli, Milano.

Morton C.H., (2002), *The (Re)-Emergence of Women-Supported Childbirth in the United States*, PhD Dissertation in Sociology, University of California.

Morton C., Clift E., (2014), *Birth Ambassadors: Doulas and the Re-Emergence of Woman-Supported Birth in America*, Praeclarus Press, Amarillo, TX.

Mosedale S., (2005), Assessing Women's Empowerment. Towards a Conceptual Framework, *Journal of International Development*, 7 (2):243–257.

Mottl-Santiago J., Walker C., Ewan J., Vragovic O., Winder S., Stubblefield P., (2008), A Hospital-Based Doula Program and Childbirth Outcomes in an Urban, Multicultural Setting, *Maternal and Child Health Journal*, 12 (3):372–377.

Najafi T.F., Roudsari L.R., Ebrahimipour H., (2017), The Best Encouraging Persons in Labor. A Content Analysis of Iranian Mothers' Experiences of Labor Support, *PLoS One*, 12 (7). https://journals.plos.org/plosone/article?id=10.1371/journal.pone.0179702.

Nommsen-Rivers L.A., Mastergeorge A.M., Hansen R.L., Cullum A.S., Dewey K.G., (2009), Doula Care, Early Breastfeeding Outcomes, and Breastfeeding Status at 6 Weeks Postpartum among Low-Income Primiparae, *Journal of Obstetric, Gynecologic, and Neonatal Nursing*, 38 (2):157–173.Oakley A., (1992), *Social Support and Motherhood. The Natural History of a Research Project*, Blackwell, Oxford.

Oakley A., Houd S., (1990), *Helpers in Childbirth. Midwifery Today*, Hemisphere Publishing Corporation, London.

OECD (2019), *Caesarean Sections (Indicator)*. DOI: 10.1787/adc3c39f-en.

Oparah J.C., James J.E., Barnett D., Jones L.M., Melbourne D., Peprah S., Walker J.A., (2021), Creativity, Resilience and Resistance: Black Birthworkers' Responses to the COVID-19 Pandemic, *Frontiers in Sociology*, 6:1–10. DOI: 10.3389/fsoc.2021.636029.

Page L., (2001), The Humanization of Birth, *International Journal of Gynecology e Obstetrics*, 75:s55–s58.

Pancino C., (1984), *Il bambino e l'acqua sporca. Storia dell'assistenza al parto dalle mammane alle ostetriche (secoli 16-19)*, Franco Angeli, Milano.

Parsons T., (1950), *The Social System*, Free Press, Glencoe, IL.

Pascali-Bonaro D., Kroeger M., (2004), Continuous Female Companionship during Childbirth: A Crucial Resource in Times of Stress or Calm, *Journal of Midwifery and Women's Health*, 49 (4):19–27.

Pasian P., (2015), La doula: l'emergere di una professione, *Autonomie Locali e Servizi sociali*, 2:291–305.

Pert C., (1997), *Molecules of Emotion: The Science behind Mind-Body Medicine*, Scribner, New York, NY.

Piazza M., (2013), Gli inciampi dell'inconscio, in Balbo L. (ed.), *Imparare, sbagliare, vivere. Storie di lifelong learning*, Franco Angeli, Milano.

Pitch T., (2006), *La società della prevenzione*, Carocci, Roma.

Pizzini F., (1985), Introduzione: il parto tra biologia e cultura, in Colombo G., Pizzini F., Regalia A., (eds.), *Mettere al mondo. La produzione sociale del parto*, Franco Angeli, Milano.

Pizzini F., (1999), *Corpo medico e corpo femminile. Parto, riproduzione artificiale, menopausa*, Franco Angeli, Milano.Pomata G., (1979), *In scienza e coscienza. Donne e potere nella società borghese*, La Nuova Italia, Firenze.

Praetorius I., (2002), La filosofia del saper esserci. Per una politica del simbolico, *Via Dogana*, 60:3–7.

Ranisio G., (1998), *Venire al mondo. Credenze, pratiche, rituali del parto*, Meltemi, Roma.

Raphael D., (1966), *Lactation, Its Biological and Cultural Confluence within the Construct of Supportive Behavior*, Unpublished PhD Dissertation, Columbia University.

Raphael D., (1969), Uncle Rhesus, Auntie Pachyderm, and Mom: All Sorts and Kinds of Mothering, *Perspectives in Biology and Medicine*, 12 (2):289–297.

Raphael D., (1973), *The Tender Gift: Breastfeeding*, Prentice-Hall, Englewood Cliffs, NJ.

Rawlings D., Litster C., Miller-Lewis L., Tieman J., Swetenham K., (2020), The Voices of Death Doulas about Their Role in End-of-Life Care, *Health and Social Care in the Community*, 28:12–21.

Regalia A., (1985), *Sapere medico e pratica istituzionale*, in Colombo G., Pizzini F., Regalia A., (eds.), *Mettere al mondo. La produzione sociale del parto*, Franco Angeli, Milano.

Riessman C.K., (1987), When Gender is Not Enough: Women Interviewing Women, *Gender and Society*, 1 (2):172–207.

Rivera M., (2021), Transitions in Black and Latinx Community-Based Doula Work in the US During COVID-19, *Frontiers in Sociology*, 6:1–8. DOI: 10.3389/fsoc.2021.611350.

Romito P., Chatelanat G., (1985), Conoscenza e controllo durante la gravidanza e il parto: come (non) si negozia il potere, in Cacciari C., Pizzini F., (eds.), *La donna paziente. Modelli di integrazione in ostetricia e ginecologia*, Unicopli, Milano.

Rothman B.K., (1982), *In Labor: Women and Power in the Birthplace*, W.W. Norton, New York, NY.

Rothman B.K., (2001), Spoiling the Pregnancy: Prenatal Diagnosis in the Netherlands, in DeVries R., Benoit C., van Teijlingen E., Wrede S., (eds.), *Birth by Design: Pregnancy, Midwifery Care and Midwifery in North America and Europe*, Routledge, New York, NY.

Rowe-Murray H.J., Fisher J.R.W., (2001), Operative Intervention in Delivery Is Associated with Compromised Early Mother-Infant Interaction, *British Journal of Obstetrics and Gynaecology*, 108:1068–1075.

Ryding E.L., Wijma B., Wijma K, (1997), Posttraumatic Stress Reaction after Emergency Cesarean Section, *Acta Obstetricia et Gynecologica Scandinavica*, 76:856–861.

Saldaña J., (2013), *The Coding Manual for Qualitative Researchers*, 2nd edition, Sage, Thousand Oaks, CA.

Saraceno C., (2003), *Mutamenti della famiglia e politiche sociali in Italia*, Il Mulino, Bologna.

Sarfatti Larson M., (1977), *The Rise of Professionalism: A Sociological Analysis*, University of California Press, Berkeley, CA.

Sargent C., Stark N., (1989), Childbirth Education and Childbirth Models. Parental Perspectives on Control, Anesthesia, and Technological Intervention in the Birth Process, *Medical Anthropology Quarterly*, 3:36–51.

Sbisà M., (1992), *Come sapere il parto. Storia, scenari, linguaggi*, Rosenberg & Sellier, Torino.

Scarpa A., (1988), *Pratiche di etnomedicina. I fattori psicosomatici nei sistemi medici tradizionali*, Red, Como.

Schinkel W., Noordegraaf M., (2011), Professionalism as Symbolic Capital: Materials for a Bourdieusian Theory of Professionalism, *Comparative Sociology*, 10:67–96.

Schroeder C., Bell J., (2005), Labor Support for Incarcerated Pregnant Women: The Doula Project, *The Prison Journal*, 85 (3):311–328.

Sciurba A., (2015), *La cura servile, la cura che serve*, Pacini, Pisa.

Sclavi M., (2003), *Arte di ascoltare e mondi possibili. Come si esce dalle cornici di cui siamo parte*, Mondadori, Milano.

Scropetta C., (2012), *Accanto alla madre. La nuova figura della doula come accompagnamento al parto e alla maternità*, Terra Nuova Edizioni, Firenze.

Sevenhuijsen S., (2000), Caring in the Third Way. The Relation between Obligation, Responsibility and Care in Third Way Discourse, *Critical Social Policy*, 20 (1):5–37.

Sevenhuijsen S., (2003), The Place of Care. The Relevance of the Feminist Ethic of Care for Social Policy, *Feminist Theory*, 4 (2):179–197.

Shlafer R.J., Hellerstedt W.L., Secor-Turner M., Gerrity E., Baker R., (2015), Doulas' Perspectives about Providing Support to Incarcerated Women: A Feasibility Study, *Public Health Nursing*, 32 (4):316–326.

Shorten A., Shorten B., Keogh J., West S., Morris J., (2005), Making Choices for Childbirth. A Randomized Controlled Trial of a Decision-Aid for Informed Birth after Cesarean, *Birth Issues in Perinatal Care*, 32:252–261.

Siebert R., (2012), *Voci e silenzi postcoloniali*, Carocci, Roma.

Simkin P., (1991), Just Another Day in a Woman's Life? Women's Long-Term Perceptions of Their First Birth Experience, *Birth*, 18:203–210.

Sosa R., Kennell J., Klaus M., Robertson S., Urrutia J., (1980), The Effect of a Supportive Companion on Perinatal Problems, Length of Labor, and Mother-Infant Interaction, *The New England Journal of Medicine*, 303 (11):597–600.

Spina E., (2009), *Ostetriche e Midwives. Spazi di autonomia e identità corporativa*, Franco Angeli, Milano.

Spina E., (2014), La professione ostetrica: mutamenti e nuove prospettive, *Cambio*, 7:53–63.

Svensson L.G., Evetts J., (eds.), (2010), *Sociology of Professions. Continental and Anglo-Saxon Traditions*, Daidalos, Goteborg.

Thachuk A., (2007), Midwifery, Informed Choice, and Reproductive Autonomy. A Relational Approach, *Feminism and Psychology*, 17:39–56.

Toffanin A.M., (2015), *Controcanto. Donne latinoamericane tra violenza e riconoscimento*, Edizioni Guerini, Milano.

Torstendahl R., Burrage M., (eds.), (1990), *The Formation of Professions. Knowledge, State and Strategy*, Sage, London.

Tousijn W., (2000), *Il sistema delle occupazioni sanitarie*, Il Mulino, Bologna.

Tousijn W., (2004), Il sistema delle occupazioni sanitarie: dominanza medica e logica professionale, *Salute e Società*, 3:52–63.

Tronto J.C., (1993), *Moral Boundaries: A Political Argument for an Ethic of Care*, Routledge, New York, NY.

Van der Hulst L.A.M., Van Teijlingen E., Bonsel G.J., Eskes M., Birnie E., Bleker O., (2007), Dutch Women's Decision-Making in Pregnancy and Labour as Seen through Eyes of Their Midwives, *Midwifery*, 23 (3):279–286. DOI: 10.1016/j.midw.2007.01.009.

Van Teijlingen E., (2005), A Critical Analysis of the Medical Model as Used in the Study of Pregnancy and Childbirth, *Sociological Research Online*, 10 (2):63–77.

Van Zandt S.E., Edwards L., Jordan E.T., (2005), Lower Epidural Anesthesia Use Associated with Labor Support by Student Nurse Doulas: Implications for Intrapartal Nursing Practice, *Complementary Therapies in Clinical Practice*, 11 (3):153–160.

Varcoe C., Brown H., Calam B., Harvey T., Tallio M., (2013), Help Bring Back the Celebration of Life: A Community-Based Participatory Study of Rural Aboriginal

Women's Maternity Experiences and Outcomes, *BMC Pregnancy Childbirth*, 13 (1):26.

Vegetti Finzi S., (1990), *Il bambino della notte. Divenire donna divenire madre*, Mondadori, Milano.

Vicarelli G., (2012), Medici e manager. Verso un nuovo professionalismo?, *Cambio*, 3:125–136.

Viciani S., (2015), Tradizione e attualità delle professioni intellettuali in Italia, in Tonarelli A., Viciani S., (eds.), *Le professioni intellettuali tra diritto e innovazione*, Pacini Editore, Pisa.

Viteritti A., (2005), *Identità e competenze. Soggettività e professionalità nella vita sociale contemporanea*, Guerini e Associati, Milano.

Who – Maternal and Newborn Health/Safe Motherhood Unit, (1996), *Care in Normal Birth: A Practical Guide*. www.who.int/maternal_child_adolescent/documents/who_frh_msm_9624/en/.

Who – UNICEF, (1989), *Protecting, Promoting and Supporting Breast-Feeding. The Special Role of Maternity Service*. www.who.int/nutrition/publications/infantfeeding/9241561300/en/.

Who – UNICEF, (2006), *Baby-Friendly Hospital Initiative*. www.who.int/nutrition/publications/infantfeeding/9789241595018/en/

Wijma K., Ryding E.L., Wijma B., (2002), Predicting Psychological Well-Being after Emergency Caesarean Section. A Preliminary Study, *Journal of Reproductive and Infant Psychology*, 20:25–36.

Wilensky H.L., (1964), The Professionalization of Everyone, *The American Journal of Sociology*, 70 (2):137–158.

Wilson S.F., Gurney E.P., Sammel M.D, Schreiber C.A., (2016), Doulas for Surgical Management of Miscarriage and Abortion: A Randomized Controlled Trial, *American Journal of Obstetrics & Gynecology*, 216 (1):44.e1–44.e6.

Witz A., (1992), *Professions and Patriarchy*, Routledge, London.

Ye J., Zhang J., Mikolajczyk R., Torloni M.R., Gülmezoglu A.M., Betrán A.P., (2016), Association between Rates of Caesarean Section and Maternal and Neonatal Mortality in the 21st Century: A Worldwide Population-Based Ecological Study with Longitudinal Data, *BJOG: An International Journal of Obstetrics & Gynaecology*, 123 (5):745–753.

Zhang J., Bernasko J.W., Leybovich E., Fahs M., Hatch M.C., (1996), Continuous Labor Support from Labor Attendant for Primiparous Women: A Meta-Analysis, *Obstetrics and Gynecology*, 88 (4):739–744.

Zola I.K., (1972), Medicine as an Institution of Social Control, *Sociological Review*, 20:487–504.

Index

For Product Safety Concerns and Information please contact our EU
representative GPSR@taylorandfrancis.com
Taylor & Francis Verlag GmbH, Kaufingerstraße 24, 80331 München, Germany

www.ingramcontent.com/pod-product-compliance
Lightning Source LLC
Chambersburg PA
CBHW060318220326
41598CB00027B/4362

9 780367 762070